ARTHRITIS:
Rational Therapy and Rehabilitation

ROBERT L. SWEZEY, M.D., F.A.C.P.

Medical Director,
The Arthritis and Back Pain Center
Santa Monica, California;

Clinical Professor of Medicine
University of California, Los Angeles;
Formerly, Chief, Division of Rehabilitation Medicine
University of California, Los Angeles

W. B. SAUNDERS COMPANY
1978 PHILADELPHIA • LONDON • TORONTO

W. B. Saunders Company: West Washington Square
Philadelphia, Pa.   19105

1 St. Anne's Road
Eastbourne, East Sussex BN21 3UN, England

1 Goldthorne Avenue
Toronto, Ontario M8Z 5T9, Canada

Arthritis: Rational Therapy and Rehabilitation   ISBN   0-7216-8690-7

Last digit is the print number: 9   8   7   6   5   4   3   2   1

To

Annette, Richard, Ken, Stuart, and *Mother*

for their thoughtfulness, love and concern, and to

Dad,

in his memory.

PREFACE

In the treatment of chronic rheumatological disorders one rarely has the opportunity to use a single therapeutic approach to the exclusion of all others. There are a number of books and review articles that detail the nature of the various rheumatological diseases and the various pharmacological and surgical approaches to them. This book will not recapitulate these aspects of rheumatological therapy but will attempt to expand on the vast array of primary and adjunctive rehabilitative therapies that supplement and, in many cases, supplant pharmacological and surgical intervention in the management of uncomplicated to complex chronic rheumatological diseases.

I have attempted to analyze what is known about the various aspects of rehabilitative treatment in rheumatic diseases and in particular I have emphasized the rationale for exercise therapy and the status of the various therapeutic modalities used for pain relief. My purpose has been to present and critically review what is known, and to develop from this the therapeutic approaches that represent a reasonable and practical synthesis so that the arthritis patient will benefit maximally from selected treatments while being encumbered as little as possible with well-intended but dubious or futile therapeutic gestures.

There are 71 illustrations designed to clarify or exemplify key aspects of various components of therapy. The book is divided into nine chapters or sections. The first chapter discusses definitions and philosophies of rehabilitation and some of the important socioeconomic issues that apply to rheumatic diseases. A description of the organization of the various components of rehabilitation treatment facilities is also provided. The second chapter reviews and discusses various aspects of the evaluation of functional loss and presents suggestions for screening and assessment of physical disability. Chapter 3 deals with the rationales for therapy and explores in depth the basis for rest, immobilization, muscle strengthening, and joint stretching. Illustrative examples of specific exercise regimens are outlined. The principles of joint protection, energy conservation, and prevention of deformity are discussed in the fourth chapter and recommendations for positioning and posture are explained and illustrated. In Chapter 5, the physiology and rationale for splinting and bracing and for casting to overcome contractures is explained and the methods discussed. Positions of function for joints where loss of motion is unavoidable are delineated. The indications and methods for splinting of a variety of common rheumatological disorders are given and specific splinting considerations for the various disorders are described. This chapter also includes commonly employed modifications of shoes, bracing for the lower extremity, and a consideration of the indications for various types of cervical collars, braces, and back supports. In Chapter 6 mobility and gait are discussed. The problems that relate to impairment of gait and the strategies used for improvement of mobility, including cane and crutch fitting, the prescription for wheelchairs, modifications of automobiles, and opportunities and problems relating to personal and public transportation, are detailed. As in all sections, references to key articles and resources are provided so that the reader can explore in whatever additional depth is desired any aspect of a problem and obtain the additional resources that might be needed to solve his patients' particular problems. Chapter 7 analyzes therapeutic modalities used for pain relief. The placebo phenomenon's impact on assessment of the efficacy of various physical agents, such as cooling and heating modalities, diathermy, and traction, as well as on the rationale for massage, manipulation, vapo coolant spray, local anesthetic injections, acupuncture, transcutaneous nerve stimulation, operant conditioning, and biofeedback is summarized. The current state of the art and of the science relating to these various modalities is explored and their role in rehabilitation therapy defined. In Chapter 8, psychological factors in rehabilitation are reviewed and the approaches, including group therapy, social intervention, and sexual counseling, are examined. The rationale for and methods and resources available to improve patient education programs and to provide recreational opportunities for patients are also presented.

Throughout these sections a great effort is made to review and condense what is of importance to comprehensive rheumatological care in these various topics and to provide a reasonable statement and basis for a choice of what is appropriate therapy based on a critical synthesis and analysis of the literature and the author's experience and judgment. The last chapter consists of 20 specific case examples selected to illustrate the practical application of the various rheumatological therapies in a variety of rheumatological problems ranging from mild rheumatoid arthritis to "trigger" fingers.

The author has spent many years practicing rheumatology and, more importantly perhaps, teaching rheumatological practice. It is hoped that this book will help to provide some answers to the many questions that arise in uncomplicated and comprehensive rheumatological-rehabilitation therapy as well as raise some significant questions for future investigations.

ROBERT L. SWEZEY, M.D.

ACKNOWLEDGMENTS

In writing this book on rheumatological rehabilitation, the author would like to underscore his debt and to express the deep gratitude that he personally and all rheumatologists interested in rehabilitation owe to Edward W. Lowman, M.D., for his leadership in identifying the rehabilitative needs of patients and the opportunities and resources to help alleviate them. I would also like to thank the UCLA Rheumatology Rehabilitation team for their assistance in the development of some of the materials and formats used in this book. In particular I would like to thank my secretaries, Mrs. Judy Katz, without whom this would never have been possible, Mrs. Lyn Charlsen, without whom it would never have been completed, and Mrs. Margaret Fansler, who tirelessly herded the loose ends of this manuscript and its author to a happy ending. I further wish to express my great appreciation to Drs. Richard Boyer, Andrea Cracchiolo, Robert Harris, Peter Kelly, Louis Kramer, Timothy Spiegel, and Lionel Walpin for their extremely helpful criticism of the contents of this book as well as for their suggestions for topics originally omitted. Mary Benz Deckert deserves great praise for her attractive illustrations, which I consider to be a major asset of this work.

Mrs. Annette Swezey has provided both important inspiration and input into the contents of this text, particularly with reference to the material on patient education, and has shown unflagging patience with the author as he struggled with the actual preparation and writing of this manuscript. To her I gratefully give my thanks and my love. I am deeply indebted to Frederic J. Kottke, M.D., who provided for me the model for critical searching inquiry into the myriad aspects of rehabilitation therapies. I also owe thanks to Dr. Daniel J. McCarty for having originally asked me to write a chapter in Arthritis and Allied Conditions which served as the final combination of inspiration and perspiration that catalyzed the genesis of this work. Last, I would like to thank the many rheumatic disease fellows, residents, interns, students, allied health professionals, and above all the patients with rheumatological diseases who have challenged me and taught me over the years. I hope that some of what I have learned will help better the lives of many other arthritis sufferers.

R.L.S.

CONTENTS

Chapter 4

JOINT PROTECTION.. 97

Chapter 5

SPLINTS, BRACES, SHOES AND CORSETS...................................... 103

LIST OF TABLES

APPENDIX

REHABILITATION AND ARTHRITIS

Definitions, Significance, Therapeutic Team and Facility Configuration

In the broadest sense, any diagnostic or therapeutic procedure that is utilized in patient evaluation and management can be considered a part of a rehabilitative process. The focus of this text will be more circumscribed and will emphasize those diagnostic and therapeutic maneuvers that are customarily — but by no means exclusively — employed and directed by physiatrists (specialists in Physical Medicine and Rehabilitation), orthopedists, and rheumatologists in the comprehensive management of disabling or potentially disabling disorders.

DEFINITIONS

A sensitivity to the distinctions between the terms impairment, handicap, and disability is essential to anyone who must involve himself in the care of chronic disease.[1] An *impairment* is a damaged, deteriorated, or injured organ or extremity, while a *handicap* is the disadvantage in function caused by the impairment. *Disability* is the inability to function effectively as a consequence of an excessive handicap resulting from an impairment. The U.S. Social Security Administration definition of disability is determined by whether the particular individual is unable to engage in any substantial gainful activity by reason of his physical or mental impairment or impairments, taking into account his age, education, and previous work experience.[2] The occupational definition, used by the Veterans Administration and many pension plans, is the finding of the lack of capability to perform

1

a previous occupation, or the percentage of disablement as judged against schedules of disability based on a presumed effect of a given condition on the "average man."[1, 3]

Given the consequences of the impairment caused by the arthritis, the challenge to the rheumatologist and to all others who treat the arthritic patient is to *minimize impairment* and *lessen the burden of the handicap* so as to *prevent disability.* An incisive definition in this connection that underlines the outstanding life successes of so many valiant people who have had arthritis is that "a handicap is a burden placed on a superior opponent in order to equalize the competition."

The specialty of Physical Medicine and Rehabilitation, which by definition and tradition has employed *physical agents* such as light, heat, water, electricity, and mechanical agents, and more recently exercise therapy (physical medicine) in the treatment and training of the patient to attain his maximum physical, psychological, social, and vocational potential for normal living (rehabilitation), has helped to emphasize the various aspects of comprehensive care in the prevention of disability. Krusen has said that, "While rehabilitation should be everybody's interest, it cannot be everybody's business."[4] For those patients who suffer from complex impairments, with various handicaps and disabilities, the efforts of highly qualified physicians and allied health professionals in various disciplines skilled in the management of the diseases they treat, integrated and orchestrated by a knowledgeable and responsible physician, are essential to a successful rehabilitation outcome.

The goals of comprehensive care for arthritic patients are to restore them to the highest possible level of function and independence that they are capable of achieving and to "enable them to obtain optimum satisfaction and usefulness in terms of themselves, their families, and their community."[4] For the arthritic patient this means maximum pain relief, restoration of mobility and strength, and above all, inculcating a sense of his value as a human being in his social setting.

SOCIAL AND ECONOMIC FACTORS IN REHABILITATION

Accountability in all aspects of human social endeavor has become an inevitable feature of any consideration of health care activities. At a time when the tax burden increases and the health care dollar takes an even larger bite of the taxpayers' contribution, accountability must now be reflected in what is called "cost effectiveness." In terms of human values the relief of pain and enhancement of an individual's independence and self image in achieving even partial restoration of participation in the opportunities and activities of society are of incalculable value to the individual, but equally impossible to calculate is the cost to society to achieve these modest goals. Commitment of national health care resources is less certain where the issues relating to the value of quality of life, preservation of function, and partial restoration of function in chronic disease are in contention with dramatic life or death considerations. An apt comparison here is that of chronic renal dialysis as a life-saving measure with on-going maintenance and restorative therapies for a multiply involved arthritic or a sufferer from other chronic neuromuscular disorders. A few examples of the economic devastation caused by rheumatic diseases are worth noting. Approximately one-third of the 3.6 million adult Americans with rheumatoid arthritis between the ages of 35 and 50 are disabled; 20 per cent of the 0.06 per cent of children under age 15 who develop juvenile rheumatoid arthritis will suffer significant crippling into adult life; approximately one million men and women over age 16 in Great Britain are disabled primarily as a consequence of rheumatic diseases; nearly one-sixth of incapacity in the industrial population of England and Wales has been attributed to rheumatic complaints.[5, 6]

It is estimated that 426.9 million dollars per annum are spent by the U.S. Veterans Administration alone on compensation for arthritis-related disability, and one billion dollars annually is spent on disability insurance payments and aid to the permanently and totally disabled.[7] In addition, "lost" homemakers' services cost $0.4 billion annually, lost wages $4.8 billion annually, and lost federal, state, and local income taxes $955 million annually.[7, 8] All these costs are in addition to the billions spent on arthritis care and rehabilitation.[8]

A number of studies of the efficacy of rehabilitation in arthritic patients have been made, and the benefits in terms of improved patient function have been shown. Less definable are the benefits when assessed in terms of cost effectiveness. Programs focused on those patients whose problems have been amenable to surgery, most notably the recipients of total hip prostheses, have been able to justify themselves on the basis of economic benefit.[5, 9-20] In a review of the economic analyses of other arthritic problems in these studies it was extremely difficult to determine cost effectiveness per se because of the variety of assumptions regarding actual costs and estimated costs and, therefore, estimated savings, tax offsets, and reduction in service requirements for therapeutic or assisting personnel, earnings lost or gained, and extrapolations based on inflationary considerations.[21]

In addition to the actuarial difficulties, it is at least as difficult to determine the merits as well as the cost effectiveness of the components of the rehabilitation therapy, including exercise, rest, splinting, occupational therapy, vocational counseling, psychological and social counseling, community support and intervention, as well as medical and surgical therapies, hospitalization costs, all intertwined with the variabilities of the natural history of the diseases themselves. Despite all the qualifications and possible assumptions and despite all the resistance by industry (even in high employment periods) to the hiring of physically handicapped, the consensus of the most critical analyses is that rehabilitation services for arthritic disorders are, in fact, cost effective and that high quality programs are likely to be accompanied by increased socioeconomic benefits to society, over and above the unaccountable benefits of pain reduction and improved psychosocial function for the arthritis sufferer.[2, 22]

It has been demonstrated that patients with major arthritic diseases are capable of effective full-time or part-time employment, but for many patients with severe involvement availability of adaptive equipment and modification of work methods as well as accessibility to a work setting are essential to successful employment.[20, 22-29] Prejudice against the handicapped worker by industry, labor unions and the insurance companies places an added burden on the handicapped or arthritic patient by restricting his opportunities for employment, thereby causing him to lose his self-esteem as well as to become an economic burden. The elimination of restrictions imposed by insurance underwriters and, in particular, provisions for softening the impact of subsequent injury contract clauses ("hold harmless" clauses) would protect industry from excessive insurance costs and would provide increased opportunity for the handicapped worker.[20, 22, 28, 29]

Although work in industry or employment in a profession are obvious goals for the physically handicapped, equally important but perhaps less widely appreciated is the role of homemaker; homemaking is now officially considered a form of employment for the blind only by the California State Department of Rehabilitation.[30] A legitimate goal of Vocational Rehabilitation and Social Security agencies is to raise the level of function of a disabled person so that he or she can be independent in homemaking activities, or require a lesser amount of supervision of personal needs or of needs for maintenance of independence in homemaking activities.[30-32] The patient who no longer requires an assistant when dressing eliminates the cost to society of providing someone to provide that assistance.[22, 27] By the same token, the patient who can do his own shopping and is independent in maintaining his household function again obviates the necessity for the cost of an additional person, full or part time, to provide those functions.[22, 28, 29]

A consideration of vocational problems is incomplete without recognition of the various occupation-related degenerative arthropathies.[33-38] These disorders, from the standpoint of prevention as well as amelioration, present a clear challenge to the industrial physician, rheumatologist, occupational therapist, vocational counselor, and to industry itself.

COMPONENTS OF THE REHABILITATION PROCESS

THE REHABILITATION THERAPEUTIC TEAM

In most instances the comprehensive care needs of the severely involved arthritic patient require the diversified skills of several of the allied health care specialties usually associated with rehabilitation centers, hospitals, and related community-supported facilities and services. The various rheumatic diseases and accompanying physical, psychological, and social derangements are best treated by physicians (rheumatologists, orthopedists, physiatrists, psychiatrists) and allied health professionals with specific training and skill in the management of rheumatological disorders. There is at this time a great deficiency of health professionals with these skills; therefore one cannot comfortably assume that a referral to a rehabilitation center which is fully manned by all appropriate allied health professions will be able to provide the expertise for management of a given rheumatic disease patient. Unfortunately, all too often the physician or surgeon refers the patient for rehabilitation therapies about which he has no knowledge to persons who are little better prepared to treat the arthritic patient. The Allied Health Professions Section of the Arthritis Foundation has taken the initiative in attempting to develop arthritis rehabilitation specialists in various allied health profession disciplines, but a great deal more needs to be accomplished within the allied health professions, and this is equally true for the medical profession itself.

THE ALLIED HEALTH PROFESSIONAL TEAM

Although most patients with arthritis and physical disability need at least some components of physical therapy and occupational therapy, the importance of any one individual in the health care team to any given patient cannot be given any priority, and indeed it is for that reason that we speak of the health care team.[39] The descriptions here of the roles of the various allied health professionals represent a customary distribution of their responsibilities, but there can be a considerable overlap from one setting to another, just as there may be between the roles of primary physicians, rheumatologists, orthopedists, and physiatrists, who with the allied health professionals constitute the full professional health care team.

The *nurse* functioning in a clinic, office, hospital, or in a visiting nurse capacity must be familiar with the various kinds of arthritic diseases, therapeutic regimens, medications, and common drug reactions. She must have the skills required to provide instruction, monitor compliance, and give support to the physically disabled patient and his or her family. She must reinforce the techniques of joint protection, energy conservation, and the continuation of prescribed therapeutic regimens.

The *occupational therapist* (O.T.) is concerned first with the patient's ability to function independently with a minimum of fatigue and of stress to the involved joints, and second with the provision of adaptive equipment to allow function that is otherwise difficult or impossible, often in conjunction with the fabrication of supporting or corrective splinting as indicated. The occupational therapist assists in teaching the patient to perform upper extremity activities in a manner least apt to cause increased inflammation or deformity. The occupational therapist may play a key role in assisting the surgeon in the postoperative management of upper extremity surgery. The occupational therapist can provide patients with activities designed and positioned to provide appropriate exercise for a variety of musculoskeletal problems, particularly where standard exercise therapy may prove boring and therefore result in compliance failures. The occupational therapist evaluates patients' life styles to help minimize their frustrations and tensions and screens the patients for their potential for work or for retraining in more appropriate occupations.

The *physical therapist* (P.T.) implements the exercise therapy program and has a particular responsibility in teaching the patient transfer and ambulation techniques. The assessment of ambulation assisting devices (cane, crutch, brace) and wheel chair needs is performed by or coordinated with the P.T. The physical therapist also administers the various modalities of therapy, including particularly heat, cold, diathermy, and traction, and instructs the patients in their home use where appropriate.

The *psychologist or psychiatrist* is often needed to assist in the management of the associated psychological problems that accompany pain and loss of function. Psychologists must be aware of the various organic psychological disorders associated with rheumatic diseases, as well as the drug-induced psychological disturbances.[40] Important in this regard is the need for the psychotherapist to be familiar with the literature relating to psychological problems in rheumatic diseases and in chronic pain syndromes in order to have an insightful approach to the psychological aspects of the arthritic patient.

The *social worker* plays an important supportive role in handling the psychological problems and family-associated dislocations that may result from the major effects of crippling and systemic rheumatic diseases. The economic stability as well as the intra-family and community relationships may become seriously disturbed and require the intervention and support of the social worker to minimize their impact.

The *vocational counselor* with an understanding of rheumatic diseases, and especially their potential for recovery and rehabilitation, can play a key role in utilizing the community and agency resources that may be essential to restore the patient to a role of active economic participation.[39]

A number of other members of the team make contributions of extreme importance.[39] The contacts of *clerical personnel* with patients may create an atmosphere of warmth, acceptance, understanding, or conversely one that is the very opposite. *Patient educators* can play a key role in bringing structured educational materials about the various diseases and the problems attendant upon their treatment to the patients and their families in a manner and in a setting designed to maximize their ability to learn and understand. *Rehabilitation counselors* can function in the interface between the social worker and the vocational counselor to provide support to the patient and his family and assist in coordinating the rehabilitation process during the time that he or she is being prepared for entry into a vocational rehabilitation program. The *volunteers* who participate in arthritis clinics or hospitals can help create a warm and compassionate milieu, especially if they have an understanding of the various arthritic diseases and their consequences. Arthritic patients can themselves play a very key role as volunteers, and this can be expanded to an ombudsman function, with a patient or concerned person providing input to the staff or administration about the arthritic patients' problems and frustrations. The most important member of the arthritis health care team is the *patient* and the second most important is the patient's family. Both must be given every opportunity to fully participate in the team deliberations and decisions.[39, 41]

The team obviously is complex and involves many disciplines and persons and personalities. There is, therefore, a constant danger of duplication of effort, waste of a specialist's time, and counterproductive efforts as a result of failure of coordination and integration of therapeutic activities.[42] An obvious example is the uncoordinated prescription of exercises for the same joint by both the physical therapist and the occupational therapist, resulting in an excessive exercise regimen for the patient and aggravation of his joint condition. Another problem is redundant psychological dabbling by sympathetic or curious health care team members where very careful integration of psychological effort is needed. The health care team must be coordinated by a responsible physician who should be sufficiently knowledgeable and involved to recognize when goals are met or are in need of revision, and who can coordinate the team in such a way that the stated goals are achieved in an expeditious manner and so that therapies no longer indicated are promptly discontinued. This highly sophisticated health care team is clearly an expensive organization, and this resource must be husbanded carefully so that each health care team member can function with maximal effectiveness and the patient's goals can be accomplished with the least effort and expense.[43]

FACILITY CONSIDERATIONS

Just as the team members differ in their skills and functions, the environment in which the rehabilitation process takes place is highly variable. The most important environment is the patient's home, but his place of work, worship, and educational and recreational facilities, in addition to the physician's office or clinic or hospital or rehabilitation facility, all potentially determine limits or opportunities for an independent life style.[42] The patient who is confined to a wheelchair is confronted with a number of problems, ranging from the impediments of curbs or stairs to narrow doorways or insufficient space in lavatories, drinking fountains too high or low, inaccessibility to most public transportation, public telephones with coin slots higher than 54 inches from the floor, and parking spaces reserved for handicapped less than 12 feet wide or located at long distances from buildings — just to mention a few. The patient who is weak or who must use canes or crutches or who ambulates with painful joints is equally impeded and must be concerned with many problems, including lengthy corridors, uneven terrain, ice, mud, heavy doors, resistant door knobs, lack of railings, and waiting room seats too low or too soft or lacking in arms needed to facilitate standing and to relieve joint stress while sitting.[44]

The actual *therapeutic facilities* (outside of the modifications to home and place of work discussed subsequently under *Joint Protection and Energy Conservation*) include the therapeutic gymnasium, hydrotherapy, and activity of daily living area or the physical therapy and occupational therapy departments, respectively. Ideally these areas should be adjacent and interrelated and in close proximity to psychological, social, and vocational counseling services.[45] Preferably the hospital rehabilitation therapy area should provide for the treatment of both inpatients and outpatients in the same location to ensure continuity of therapy and to minimize the redundancy of reevaluation and treatment by a second therapist not familiar with either the patient or his prior regimen.

The *therapeutic gymnasium* adequate for a small hospital requires about 375 square feet (34.8 meters^2) and should include an exercise mat (preferably raised for easier access), a plinth or exercise table, parallel bars, and corner stairs for gait training, a full-length mirror and an area for cervical traction. Space for a shoulder wheel and finger ladder and reciprocal pulleys is desirable. Additional space for a Hubbard tank (ideally a therapeutic pool) as well as for a whirlpool is requisite. Treatment areas for application of paraffin, diathermy, and ultrasound and additional plinths for physical examinations add flexibility to the treatment area. For group physical therapy, increased mat space is required and a large therapeutic pool is desirable. Provision of a heavy duty overhead wired grid for a variety of pulley attachments provides flexibility where traction, reciprocal pulleys, or supporting slings are needed. Storage space for walkers, wheelchairs, gurneys, canes and crutches, mats, weights, and other equipment must be provided. A hydraulic lift can facilitate transfer in a variety of settings. Additional space permits the use of more elaborate equipment such as the standing tilt table for postural conditioning and gravity-assisted stretching, or a padded and adjustable table containing cables to which graded increments of weights can be attached (a De Lorme or Elgin exercise table) to facilitate the design of a variety of stretching or isotonic strengthening regimens.[46] (See *Strengthening Exercises* in Chapter 3.)

Indoor therapeutic pools can be as small as 2 x 3 meters (6 x 9 feet) with a maximum depth of 1.5 meters and a minimum depth of 1 meter (0.75 meter for children). The maximum practical pool size for a medical facility is 5 x 8 meters. The floor of the pool is best flat or terraced with 10 to 15 cm. steps between levels. If sloped, the pool's floor should not exceed seven degrees. Hubbard tank dimensions are approximately 2 x 3 meters. Some Hubbard tanks have a grating at the base which can be removed to allow the patient to stand supported in water at optimal depths to permit ambulation training where weight bearing must be minimized.[47] Transfer to and from the non-ambulatory patient's litter to the Hubbard tank or pool is facilitated by means of electrically driven overhead cranes. Small tanks for finger or hand exercises can be provided although a suitable basin should serve this purpose. It must be remembered that provision of space for gurneys or wheelchairs and for therapist access around pool or tank facilities must be made. Finally, space must be provided for dressing rooms, lavatories, storage, and for cleaning and sterilization equipment and procedures.[47]

The *occupational therapy* area serves as the base for evaluation of activities of daily living (ADL). Much of this evaluation, such as bathroom and chair transfers, feeding, toileting, and personal grooming, can be performed at the patient's bedside, but it is usually more efficient to provide for these evaluations in the occupational therapy treatment area. Although specific activities, such as preparation of food and performance of household tasks (sweeping, cleaning, laundering, cooking), can be simulated, it is preferable to provide selected items of household equipment and appliances in the occupational therapy area to permit adequate testing and training of patients in joint protection and energy conservation as well as to illustrate adaptations or suitable rearrangements for their home.

Provision of a small counter and storage area should be made for splint fabrication and testing. A work bench or table used for patient evaluations or for therapeutic exercise training should have wheelchair access and preferably an adjustable table height capability. Sinks constructed to permit wheelchair proximity, and provisions for overhead sling support for weak upper extremities are needed. Office space for the therapists and assistants and space for privacy for individual ADL evaluation, counseling, and training should be provided.[45] Ideally, occupational therapy and physical therapy should be adjacent and located in close proximity to the patients' beds and the nursing staff to maximize team interaction and reinforcement of treatment programs. Provisions for prevocational assessment, including simulated factory, office, or outdoor physical labor or driving assessment and training, are useful extensions of occupational therapy functions but largely applicable to major rehabilitation facilities.

Socialization areas are important features of a rehabilitation facility. These include group dining and education and recreation spaces designed to accommodate wheelchairs and stretchers. There should be room for group discussions and privacy for family visits or counseling. In light of the importance of sexuality to disability associated with musculoskeletal disorders (See *Psychological Factors in Rehabilitation* in Chapter 8), it would be highly desirable to provide suitable facility arrangements and privacy for conjugal visitations. The Title 22 Health Facilities and Referral Agencies Regulations for licensing of rehabilitation centers under Social Security stipulates that such facilities must provide comprehensive services in an environment free of architectural barriers and designed with space allocated to medical diagnosis and treatment, implementation of all major allied health professional services, dining, socialization, outdoor access, recreation, and education.[32]

SELECTED READINGS BY TOPICS

(See also complete Bibliography on page 213.)

Social and Economic Factors

4. Krusen, F. H., Kottke, F. J., Ellwood, P. M., eds.: *Handbook of Physical Medicine and Rehabilitation*, 2nd Ed. Philadelphia: W. B. Saunders Co., 1971.
5. Nuki, G., Brooks, R., Buchanan, W. W.: The economics of arthritis. Bull. Rheum. Dis., *23*:(8–9):726, Series 1972–1973.
17. Duff, I. F., Carpenter, J. O., Neukom, J. E.: Comprehensive management of patients with rheumatoid arthritis. Some results of the regional arthritis control program in Michigan. Arthritis Rheum., *17*(4):635, 1974.
18. Vignos, P. J., Jr., et al.: Comprehensive care and psycho-social factors in rehabilitation in chronic rheumatoid arthritis: a controlled study. J. Chronic Dis., *25*:457, Aug. 1972.
19. Acheson, R. M., Crago, A., Weinerman, E. R.: New Haven survey of joint diseases. Institutional and social care for the arthritic. J. Chronic Dis., *23*:843, May 1971.
20. Robinson, H. S.: "Prognosis: Return to work — Arthritis," *in* G. E. Ehrlich, ed., *Total Management of the Arthritic Patient*. Philadelphia: J. B. Lippincott Co., 1973. P. 183.
21. Nuki, G., Brooks, R., Buchanan, W. W.: *Bulletin on Rheumatic Diseases and Disability Insurance*. Legislative issue paper prepared by the staff on the Subcommittee on

Social Security. Washington: U. S. Government Printing Office, May 1976. P. 28.

24. Karten, I., Lee, M., McEwen, C.: Rheumatoid arthritis: five-year study of rehabilitation. Arch. Phys. Med. Rehabil., *54*:120, Mar. 1973.

The Rehabilitation Therapeutic Team

39. Leviton, G. L.: "Professional-client relations in a rehabilitation hospital setting," *in* W. S. Neff, ed., *Rehabilitation Psychology*. Washington, D.C.: American Psychological Association, Inc., 1971. P. 215.
43. Halstead, L. S.: Team care in chronic illness. A critical review of the literature of the past 25 years. Arch. Phys. Med. Rehabil., *57*:507, Academy Issue, Nov. 1976.

Facility Considerations

45. Erickson, E. R., Pedersen, E.: Design criteria for a rehabilitation unit. Hospitals, *39*:53, Mar. 1965.
46. Boyle, R. W.: "Chapter 9. The therapeutic gymnasium," *in* S. Licht, ed., *Therapeutic Exercise*. New Haven: Elizabeth Licht, 1961. P. 257.
47. Stewart, J. B.: "Chapter 10. Exercises in water." *in* S. Licht, ed., *Therapeutic Exercise*. 2nd Ed. Baltimore: Waverly Press. 1965. P. 285.

Chapter 2 _____

EVALUATION OF FUNCTION

EVALUATION OF DISABILITY

As defined, a physical disability has a socio-economic as well as physical and psychological component. In order to measure a physical disability one has to be able to quantify function and levels of lack of function. This must be differentiated from the quantification of pain (discussed in Chapter 7, *Therapeutic Modalities for Pain Relief*) or loss of mobility (discussed under *Stretching Exercises* in Chapter 3), or loss of strength (discussed under *Strengthening Exercises* in Chapter 3). The purpose of a functional evaluation is to describe and quantify levels of functional impairment and independence in various activities. This quantification is essential for optimal selection of work levels and housing or for the determination of the level of supervision in nursing care that a given patient may require. It is equally important to quantify function in order to measure the effectiveness of therapeutic interventions. Improvement of function in most instances rates second only to relief of pain as a therapeutic objective. The effort required to increase the range of motion in a given joint, in terms of expense, time, and discomfort to the patient, should be justifiable in terms of concomitant improvement in function or relief of pain.[48, 49]

Galen is given credit for adding the loss of function as an evaluative criteria to the four classic signs of inflammation.[50] More recently (1937) Taylor discussed the evaluation of function in rheumatoid arthritis, dividing degrees of impairment into slight, moderate, severe, and extreme.[50, 51] Although Taylor's classification was admirable in its brevity, it did not gain wide acceptance. A variety of evaluative formats, including testing procedures for range of motion and strength and comprehensive tests of daily living functions, continue to be employed because they have proved to be useful in the evaluation and management of specific patients and specific problems. Nonetheless, their length, detail, and the lack of validation of their scoring procedures preclude their general use.[52-54]

A *functional evaluation for arthritis* and related musculoskeletal dysfunctions must be concise, reproducible, inexpensive, and quick to administer, and preferably objective. It should distinguish upper from lower extremity dysfunctions but not ignore the head, neck, and trunk. It will be affected by pain and psychological factors but should not be a measure of them per se. Intelligence, gross behavioral disorders, and bowel and bladder continence are considerations that are appropriately evaluated in many physical disabilities, including the CNS manifestations of vasculitis, but unduly complicate any effort to make a concise statement about disability as a consequence of rheumatic disease related musculoskeletal dysfunction.

A functional test cannot and should not substitute for tests of precise mobility and strength, anatomical or radiographic descriptions, or attempts at quantification of pain and inflammation, but should be capable of reflecting the use of all major joint areas in normal daily activity tests, so that failure to perform a specified function will detect some physical deficit, and no important physical or functional deficit will go unnoticed.[55] A patient's functional inability to pick up a key to open a door may reflect loss of sensation, impaired index finger or thumb function in one or several joints, or muscular weakness of the relevant muscles, but only the functional deficit would be noted and further specific evaluation to delineate the basis for the functional loss would be required. Nonetheless, treatment designed to improve function (carpal tunnel release, splinting of thumb, or exercise of intrinsic muscles) would reflect improvement if the patient subsequently could pick up the key.

There are several purposes that a functional evaluation may serve and each purpose may require a different kind of evaluation in terms of its length, diversity, and complexity. The choices of criteria for function measurement will be determined by the settings in which an interview or questionnaire or tests of function are performed and by how well the specific measurement objectives of the proposed tests relate to the problem under study. Evaluations of specific anatomical regions or limited therapeutic interventions and objectives, such as evaluations of pre- and postoperative hand function, require appropriately specific measures of function.[56-67]

The bases for deciding what items to include in a functional evaluation, what degree of performance of each item is necessary to determine a functional level, and how many levels of function are necessary to adequately discriminate between varying degrees of disability are arbitrary, and the varieties of scoring systems that have been developed are testimony to the difficulty in achieving a consensus.[50, 52, 53, 66-86] Function tests may be insufficient in detail or suffer from redundancy. The patient's ability to perform one task can serve as a measure for a number of related tasks, e.g., picking up a key requires fingertip sensation and coordination of the thumb to the index fingertip. Testing further by picking up coins, matchsticks, pins, or chips may add nothing to the "key" test. The lack of tip pinch may not obviate the ability to pick up a key in actual practice, however, since the patient may learn to compensate by sliding the key across and off the table top into his hand.

The "functional" measures originally incorporated in the American Rheumatism Association Standard Data Base for Rheumatic Disease, including only the Steinbrocker classification (Table 2–1), grip strength, the 50-foot walking time, and a description of gait, have been significantly expanded to include descriptors of compliance, sexual functions, and upper and lower extremity activities including self-care.[87-89] This represents a major advance in institutionalizing functional testing but lacks sufficient sensitivity and specificity for many test situations. Finally, what one can measure as "function" under institution test conditions may not be used as function in actuality.[48-49] A patient may demonstrate ability to comb her hair but in fact arrange to have others do it.

Table 2–1 shows the two most widely used short functional evaluation classifications for rheumatic diseases. Both these classifications have won wide acceptance because of their brevity and succinctness and because of their similarity to the already established classification of the American Heart Association Classification for Cardiac Disease. The difficulty with these criteria is their lack of refinement. They do not distinguish primary upper from lower extremity problems and do not reflect modest but useful gains in function. For example, a patient with degenerative joint disease in one hip may be a Steinbrocker III and following surgery become a Steinbrocker II, and although signifi-

TABLE 2-1. Functional Criteria

American Rheumatism Association (U.S.A.)
1. Performs all usual activities without handicaps.
2. Performs adequately for normal activities, despite discomfort occasionally in one or more joints.
3. Limited to little or no activities or usual occupation or self-care.
4. Largely or wholly incapacitated, bed-ridden, or confined to wheelchair, little or no self-care.[80]

Joint Committee (Great Britain)

Grade 1. Fully employed or employable in the usual work and able to undertake normal physical recreation.

Grade 2. Doing light or part-time work and only limited physical recreation. For housewives, all except the heaviest housework.

Grade 3. Not employed and unemployable. No physical recreations. Housewives, only light housework and limited shopping.

Grade 4. Confined to house or wheelchair, but able to look after oneself and essentials of life. Hospital patients confined to bed.

Grade 5. Completely bedridden.[69]

cant subsequent improvement in strength and endurance and in dressing and grooming occur, he may still remain a Steinbrocker II.[80]

Notable efforts to resolve some of these conflicts include the functional classification of the Rancho Los Amigos Hospital Physical Therapy Department in California, the classification by H. A. Smythe in his Assessment of Joint Disease, the PULSES formula of Eugene Moskowitz, et al., and the "Initial General Rating" of Redford.[90-93] The latter proposal is more inclusive in that sensory deficits, excretory function, and mental and emotional status as well as general physical condition are included, but none of these classifications are sufficiently refined or sensitive to describe succinctly levels of functional impairments and still identify important changes in function. A proposal for an abbreviated functional assessment which distinguishes upper extremity (self-care) from lower extremity (mobility) is presented in Table 2–2 as an alternative to the Steinbrocker classification.[80]

TABLE 2–2. Proposed Abbreviated Functional Disability Classification

A. *Upper Extremity:* (Self-care and communication) Includes feeding, grooming, toileting, bathing, dressing, typing or writing, and telephoning.
    1. *Normal:* Can perform all activities efficiently and at a level compatible with normal recreational and vocational needs.
    2. *Independent:* Performs all activities without assistance or assistive devices but may have some discomfort, awkwardness, or inefficiency in accomplishing task.
    3. *Partially independent:* Requires assistive devices or special preparation or scheduling of activities because of pain, weakness, fatigue, or limitation of motion.
    4. *Partially dependent:* Requires assistance or supervision in some activities.
    5. *Dependent:* Requires assistance or supervision in most functions.

B. *Lower Extremity:* (Mobility) Includes walking indoors and outdoors, up and down stairs; transferring from supine to sitting and sitting to standing, to tub or toilet; bending, moving in bed, operating a wheelchair or automobile.
    1. *Normal:* Can perform all activities efficiently and at a level compatible with normal recreational and vocational needs.
    2. *Independent:* Performs all activities without assistance or assistive devices but may have some discomfort, awkwardness, or inefficiency in accomplishing task.
    3. *Partially independent:* Requires an aid such as a cane, crutch, or walker, or is unable to handle irregular terrain, steps, prolonged walking or standing, or certain architectural barriers, or has difficulty transferring from a low seated position.
    4. *Partially dependent:* Requires a wheelchair, or assistance in some transfers, or practical ambulation is restricted to household.
    5. *Dependent:* Bedridden or requires assistance with most transfers.

EXPANDED FUNCTIONAL EVALUATION

The obvious limitations of brief functional evaluations are that they do not permit identification of the anatomical area responsible for a specific functional deficit. Was the deficit in self-care (hair combing) due to hand weakness or shoulder dysfunction? Because of the excessive time required to perform the traditional comprehensive activity of daily living (ADL) evaluation or the specific focus of certain

TABLE 2–3. Functional Evaluation[50]

---

1. Can you turn your head from side to side?
2. Can you comb your hair (at the back of your head)?
3. Can you close drawers (with arms only)?
4. Can you open doors?
5. Can you lift a full teapot?
6. Can you lift a cup with one hand and drink with it?
7. Can you turn a key in a lock?
8. Can you cut meat with a knife?
9. Can you butter bread?
10. Can you wind a watch?
11. Can you walk?
12. Can you walk without   (a) someone's help?
                             (b) crutches?
                             (c) a walking stick?
13. Can you walk up a flight of stairs?
14. Can you walk down a flight of stairs?
15. Can you stand up with your knees straight?
16. Can you stand on your toes?
17. Can you bend down to pick something up off the floor?

The answers are scored: 0 = Yes, with no difficulty;
                              1 = Yes, but with difficulty, e.g., pain, weakness, or stiffness.
                              2 = No.

---

functional evaluations, such as the Functional Life Scale or evaluations for vocational purposes, there have been a number of efforts made to develop a reasonably comprehensive yet practical functional evaluation that meets the criteria of simplicity, economy, and reproducibility.[50, 52, 53, 66, 68, 70-79, 81-84, 94-100] The variety ·of attempts attests to the lack of complete acceptance of any one method.

The Functional Assessment of Polyarticular Disability from the University of California at San Diego and the Functional Index of Lee et al., from Glasgow, involve interview techniques and utilize structured questionnaires.[50, 76] Both have been subjected to careful evaluation from the standpoint of reproducibility and inter and intra-observer error and have been found to be highly reproducible, but rely on *subjective assessments*.[50, 76] (See Table 2–3.)

The problem of weighting the values attributed to each level of function in any scoring system is that there is no agreed upon measure of the degree of difficulty in the tasks listed. An objective test scoring gross movements or exercises as representative measures of function has been validated.[85] The *objective test* that has the greatest acceptance is the Barthel Index. It assesses the same spectrum of functional items found in most functional tests but includes ratings of bowel and bladder function and wheelchair manipulation, which are less commonly scored in arthritis rehabilitation.[75] Granger and Greer have attempted to define functional levels in the Barthel Index more precisely by including these measurement criteria: independent with two subcategories, intact and limited and dependent with two subcategories, helper and null or unable.[75] Granger further incorporates a gross evaluation of active motion of the right upper and left upper limbs and right lower and left lower limbs, and his evaluation requires a fairly extensive inquiry into the patient's total life functional status.[75] These criteria are too extensive in some categories and insufficient in others for rheumatological patients, but like the ARA data base they have the advantage of being designed for computerization and permit ongoing evaluation of clinical status change.

A simplified but objectively scored functional evaluation involving routine items similar to those in the questionnaire used by Lee et al. and designed so that each task is representative of a sufficiently wide range of activities to detect musculoskeletal deficits in all major areas of function is presented in Table 2–4.[50] Although this efficient format for evaluation of musculoskeletal function in arthritis meets most of the theoretical concerns, it does not include social, psychological, and vocational activity scales. Validation of its reproducibility, specificity, and selectivity as a descriptor of functional change must, however, await further study.

In addition to the need to develop a shorthand method for categorizing functional disability that is readily utilizable by physicians and a more comprehensive technique for quantifying functional deficits, there is also a need for a *shorthand screening evaluation* which will permit the physician or allied health professional to rapidly detect functional deficits in order to ensure that appropriate therapy will be carried out. The use of a screening questionnaire which can be administered by office or clinic staff for new patients helps identify many problems needing therapy. (See Table 2–5, screening form.)

Perhaps the easiest way for the physician or health professional to remember to ask the appropriate questions is to relate them to his patient's personal daily schedule as suggested below:

Starting the day: Inquiry should be made about getting out of bed, getting on and off the toilet, bathing, showering, washing teeth, caring for dentures, shaving, grooming, relating to bowel and bladder function, taking medicine, reading labels and opening medicine bottles. Functions associated with dressing, such as putting on undergarments including bras, buttoning buttons, putting on stockings or trousers, tying shoes, and donning braces and splints can be inventoried. Difficulties encountered at breakfast in preparation of food and eating, as well as any difficulties encountered in transfer into and out of chairs or washing the dishes, sweeping, and making the bed, should be sought.

Problems related to *work and homemaking* include: ambulation, ability to walk steps in and out of the house or in and out of the place of work, driving, getting in and out of a car and on or off public transportation conveyances, and use of ambulation assistive devices, wheelchairs, canes, and crutches needed to carry out the work or household tasks.

TABLE 2–4. Proposed Brief Objective Evaluation of Functional Ability

Place a check ($\checkmark$) in the appropriate column to designate the patient's level of performance. Use the following guidelines to determine the level of performance.

INDEPENDENT (I): The patient is able to initiate the activity and complete it without the assistance of another *person* or the use of an assistive device within a practical amount of time. Score (I) = 0.

INDEPENDENT WITH DEVICE (ID): The patient requires assistive device for independence, e.g., splint, brace, crutch, specially modified utensil. Score (ID) = 1

DEPENDENT (D): The patient is able to perform only part of the activity and requires the assistance of another *person*, with or without a device, to initiate or complete the activity. Score (D) = 2.

UNABLE (U): The patient cannot or will not attempt to perform the activity or cannot or will not perform any part of it when assisted by another person. Score (U) = 3.

If the patient performs the activity independently or with assistance but requires more than a practical amount of time to complete it, insert the letter "S" (slowly) in the appropriate column and add 1 to the score in columns (1), (ID), or (D).

	(1)	(ID)	(D)	(U)	COMMENTS
1. Butter bread					
2. Pick up key from table top					
3. Insert and turn key in door					
4. Open 3-inch lidded jar					
5. Pick up full glass of water and take drink					
6. Put on pullover garment					
7. Put on cardigan (blouse or shirt)					
8. Put on/take off socks/stockings					
9. Tie or fasten shoes					
10. Brush/comb hair (reaching all areas)					
11. Turn on/off light switch					
12. Use telephone (dial standard phone)					
13. Turn over and sit up in bed					
14. Get on and off toilet					
15. Get down on floor and up again					
16. Walk up 5 steps 7–8 inches high					
17. Walk down 5 steps 7–8 inches high					
18. Gait*					
SUBTOTALS:					
TOTALS:					

*Gait Score: (1) = no cane   (ID) = Cane or Crutch   (D) = 2 crutches or Walker
    (U) = Wheelchair or Unable
Timed 50 foot walk, in seconds_____

TABLE 2–5. Rheumatic Disease Self-Assessment of Function

Dear patient,

   In order to help us learn whether you will need therapy in addition to the medicine prescribed for you, please fill out this form.

DIAGNOSIS: _____ Don't know _____

USUAL VOCATION (housewife, carpenter, etc.): _____ EMPLOYED?_____Yes _____ No

IF NOT EMPLOYED, retired? _____ on disability? _____

Please check (✔) the best answer for you.

HOW MUCH PAIN and/or DIFFICULTY (stiffness, weakness, loss of balance) DO YOU HAVE WITH THE FOLLOWING ACTIVITIES?	AMOUNT			FREQUENCY	
	None	Some	Much	Some-times	Usually
1. EATING:					
cutting meat, drinking from a cup, etc.					
2. DRESSING:					
arms & upper part of body					
legs & lower part of body					
fastening buttons, zippers or snaps					
3. GENERAL HAND ACTIVITIES:					
using key, writing, dialing phone					
opening jars, drawers or doors					
4. LIFTING:					
holding objects					
bending to pick up objects					
5. PERSONAL HYGIENE:					
brushing teeth, combing hair, shaving					
toileting after-care (wiping, washing, etc.)					
6. MOBILITY:					
getting on and/or off toilet					
getting into and/or out of chair					
bed					
car					
tub					
shower					
walking inside home					
walking outside home					
walking up and/or down stairs					
7. HOME ACTIVITIES:					
gardening					
housekeeping					
cooking					
laundry					
8. ANY OTHER ACTIVITIES?					

9. How TIRED ARE YOU after an average day's activity? slightly_____ moderately_____ extremely_____ not at all _____

10. Do you perform any HOME EXERCISE PROGRAM? Yes_____ No_____

   If YES, was it prescribed by a doctor or therapist? Yes_____ No_____

11. Check any of the following which you *presently* use: splints_____ canes or crutches _____ wheelchair_____ other aids_____ none_____

12. What is your usual means of TRANSPORTATION? drive self_____ driven by family or friend _____ public transportation (taxi, bus, or van) _____

COMMENTS: _____

Problems related to financial security and employment and *psychosocial considerations* in connection with recreation, interpersonal relations, or sex should be considered. The habit of making these inquiries is readily reinforced by the needs that are identified and by the potential for successfully solving so many of the problems that plague arthritic patients.[101]

SELECTED READINGS BY TOPICS

(See also complete Bibliography on page 213.)

Evaluation of Functions

75. Granger, C. V., Greer, D. S.: Functional status measurement and medical rehabilitation outcomes. Arch. Phys. Med. Rehabil., 57(3):103, 1976.
78. Robinson, H. S., Bashall, D. A.: "Functional assessment," *in* G. E. Ehrlich, ed., *Total Management of the Arthritic Patient.* Philadelphia: J. B. Lippincott Co., 1973. P. 241.
89. Hess, E. V.: A uniform database for rheumatic diseases. Prepared by the Computer Committee of the American Rheumatism Association. Arthritis Rheum., 19:645, May–Jun. 1976.

Chapter 3

RATIONALES AND METHODS IN EXERCISE THERAPY

Stretching Exercises, Strengthening Exercises, Endurance Exercises, Specific Exercises for Specific Problems

The term exercise evokes a variety of images. "Getting exercise" can mean jogging for miles, lifting weights, or playing croquet. From the standpoint of rehabilitation, exercise therapy (over and above the psychosocial and physiological benefits of recreation) is designed to achieve specific therapeutic goals. These goals may be to maintain joint motion, increase mobility, maintain strength, or increase strength, and, ultimately, to improve function. The rationale for the specific design of a therapeutic exercise is determined by exercise physiology considerations and by the limitations of functions imposed by the damaging effects of the musculoskeletal disease, or the consequences of its therapy (e.g., steroid myopathy).

REST AND RELAXATION IN EXERCISE

It is well established that absolute bed rest has no place in the management of arthritic disorders, but selective rest or immobilization of affected joints and adequate general rest can induce a significant subsidence of inflammatory joint disease.[102-105] The debilitating physical and psychological effects of bed rest are well known, and the danger of joint ankylosis due to immobilization has long been recognized. Therefore, it is important to appreciate that immobilization (even of inflamed joints) for as long as four weeks can be accomplished without significant loss of joint mobility although a diminution of strength due to disuse is inevitable.[106-110]

Because of the additional mechanical stress imposed on abnormal joints by faulty *posture,* considerations of *prophylactic rest positions* in bed for preventing hip flexion contractures, or rest in the form of modification of activities to protect a painful back from stress, for example, are of critical importance.[111-113] (See *Posture Position and Body Mechanics* in Chapter 4.) Postural stresses must be considered in the context of functional activities (lifting and reaching during housework) as well as in the design of therapeutic exercises.

Posture and position play a major role in *relaxation.* Stretching exercises (discussed subsequently) cannot be effectively performed without relaxation of the muscles overlying the joints to be stretched. In our tense society, the need for general muscular relaxation has become widely recognized and techniques to teach this may help to permit a very tense patient to relax and, even more specifically, prepare him for stretching exercises and postural training.[114-116] Further, techniques that employ brief contractions of agonist muscles to induce reflex relaxation of antagonists (contract-relax or rhythmic stabilization exercises) can augment assisted stretching to increase range of motion of affected joints, particularly in the neck and shoulder as well as in other large proximal joints.[117-120] (See Fig. 17.)

STRETCHING EXERCISES

The purpose of stretching exercises is to prevent contracture or to increase range of motion where contracture has occurred. Evidence suggesting that exercise has reversed deformity associated with over-stretched ligaments (e.g., realigning subluxated joints) is unconvincing.[121] Contractures can be enhanced by faulty posture or position of joints and appropriate measures must be taken to prevent malpositioning. The patient with an arthritic knee who places a pillow behind it to put the joint in a position of mid-range and maximum comfort risks the development of a knee flexion contracture, a hip flexion contracture, and because of the plantar flexed position of the foot, a flexion contracture of the ankle as well as an associated shortening of the gastrocnemius-soleus musculotendinous linkage.

In addition to posture instruction and such measures as prone positioning for the patient at risk of developing hip flexion contractures, seating adjustments, work height arrangements, and supportive splinting or bracing may be required as preventive posture control measures. Where only posture is employed to prevent contractures and joint mobility is not additionally encouraged, contractures may still occur, albeit in positions more consistent with useful function. Therefore, it is essential to put all joints through a range of motion once daily if mobility is to be preserved. To attain the goal of increased joint mobility specific stretching techniques must be chosen to avoid aggravation of joint pain and inflammation.

In order to better understand the rationale for stretching exercises, it is important to recognize that joint contractures involve the joint capsule, the synovium, ligaments, and the adjacent muscles.[122-128] The looseness of the "weave" of the collagen fibers and the thickness of the individual strands in fascia, joint capsules, ligaments, or tendons vary according to the tissue structure and its function. The loose irregular weave and delicate fibers of areolar tissue contrasts with the roughly oriented coarse fibers of heavy ligaments and the highly oriented parallel fibers of many tendons. The fiber interdigitations in the fabric of fascia capsules and ligaments are potential points for adhesion formation when normal movement is restricted.[127, 128] Ligamentous and capsular structures (as well as skin) are also prestressed and therefore tend to shorten when normal tissue tension or stretching forces are interrupted.[129-131] A proximal interphalangeal joint undergoing hyperextension deformity (swan's neck) will ultimately develop tightening of its dorsal capsular fibers.[13] (See Fig. 1.)

In the arthritic patient contractures can occur in noninvolved joints as a consequence of disturbed postural mechanisms, although they typically occur because of responses to protective mechanisms associated with avoidance of painful stimuli that result from active joint disease.[133] An important additional mechanism in the genesis of joint contractures is the presence of synovial effusions. A mild or modest effusion may have very little effect on the mobility of the joint in a patient whose capsular structures are lax (although stretching of the capsule may lead to instability of the joint), but in a patient whose capsular structures tend to be less yielding the presence of fluid within the synovial space will serve as a mechanical restriction to motion. It is clear that efforts to remove effusions and to minimize recurrence of effusion are of importance in such circumstances if contractures are to be avoided.

Both joint capsular structures and muscle per se will undergo adaptive shortening during immobilization even in the absence of any inflammatory process.[122] There is evidence that these contractures occur largely due to the loss of glycosaminoglycans which may permit increased cross-linking between existing collagen fibers in both joint capsular structures and synovial tissues.[122] It has been suggested that joint mobility precludes the development of anomalous cross-links by stimulating proteoglycan synthesis, which in turn maintains a critical distance between existing collagen fibers, orders the position of new fibers, and prevents stationary fiber-to-fiber interaction and linkage.[122] In the presence of joint inflammation, connective tissue breakdown is stimulated by the collagenolytic activity of synovial enzymes, and this process and the attendant edema tend to impair joint movement and increase connective tissue turnover and remodeling and thus enhance the development of contractures.[134-136]

There are several important considerations that stem from the pathophysiological factors relating to the stretching of connective tissue in arthritics. First, with a slowly increasing tension, connective tissue tends to deform gradually up to the point of rupture, whereas a lesser force applied abruptly would cause an early rupture.[129-131] Second, collagen is more susceptible to collagenase activity (and disruption of molecular bonds) when stretched and when heated.[137, 138] Third, repetitive movement will aggravate the inflammatory and, hence, the destructive enzymatic process in inflamed joints.[128, 135, 137-141] A consideration of these factors helps determine the approach necessary to minimize the ultimate problems of loss of joint mobility and function.

METHODS FOR STRETCHING

Serial casting, progressive corrective splinting, and traction are techniques that permit prolonged gentle forces to cause a gradual "plastic" deformation and stretch. (See Figs. 24, 26, and 28.) When successful, these techniques can obviate the need for surgical release of contractures. They are best applied in patients with moderate contractures. Joint effusions should be removed or diminished by aspiration and local steroid injections prior to or during the course of these procedures. Care to prevent subluxing stresses is essential if serial or wedged casts are applied. One can anticipate a gain of about five degrees a week with serial casting for knee contractures, and traction is usually more efficient.[128, 142-146] Dynamic splinting, in which constant low grade tension creates a corrective force, can be used in selected stretching therapies. Examples of this are the use of spring and rubber band tension–activated splint devices, or webbed belts wound so that they create a low-grade dynamic tension to correct contracture deformities of a finger or elbow.[128, 142-144, 147-152] (See Figs. 7 and 8.)

PRECAUTIONS AND GENERAL CONSIDERATIONS

Exercises to increase range of motion must be graded according to the degree of inflammation and particularly according to pain tolerance. In order to minimize exacerbations of arthritis, *exercises should be performed in such a manner that any exercise-induced pain will subside within two hours or any prolonged exacerbation of pain that has occurred from exercise should have largely subsided by the following day.* Exercises must be designed and performed so as to cause the least possible stress to the joints. This means that *the fewest possible movements done in the least stressful manner possible to accomplish the goal* are objectives of the design of stretching exercise therapy.

As a general rule, the patient will require several "warm-up" movements before an optimal stretch can be made, but once the joint has been taken through its maximal range of motion (which might require anywhere from three to ten efforts), that single exercise session is usually sufficient to *maintain joint mobility* for that day.[153-157] Where the goal of stretching exercises is to *increase joint mobility,* the same precautions previously mentioned apply, but the exercise can be repeated more often (three to ten exercise sessions per day), provided increased pain and inflammation do not occur.

In patients with active rheumatoid disease and other disorders associated with morning stiffness or the "gel" phenomenon, stretching exercises designed to maintain optimal motion should be performed at the time when the "gel" phenomenon is at its least. This does not preclude the patient's performing a loosening up routine to provide sufficient mobility to start his day, but it does mean that *the major exercise effort, both for stretching and strengthening, should be done at a time when he is at his best.* This often requires the use of preliminary hot applications or a warm bath or shower, and medication, both anti-inflammatory and analgesic, taken so as to be maximally effective at the time of exercise.

Stretching exercises are characterized as passive, assisted, or active. In acute inflammation or in the presence of paralysis or mechanical joint derangement, purely passive exercise may be required to preserve or increase joint motion.[111] (See Figs. 2 to 4.) More often the patient can initiate partial movement and requires assistance to complete the exercise (active-assisted). (See Figs. 9, 15, 21, 25, and 27.) As the disease subsides, simple assistive devices, such as reciprocal pulleys, can be used in active-assisted exercises. For example, the "good arm" can pull down on one end of a rope suspended by a pulley to assist a contractured shoulder to stretch upward into forward flexion.[111] (See Fig. 13.)

Positioning a patient so that desired movement takes place in a horizontal plane eliminates the stress of gravity and may permit a better stretching motion (Figs. 10, 20). In some situations, most notably the Codman shoulder exercise, the patient can lean forward with the shoulder and arm hanging so that gravity actually assists rotary movements of the shoulder.[158] (See Fig. 12.) The warmth and buoyancy of water, particularly in a pool, may be of valuable assistance in many stretching regimens.[159] Active exercises are usually best employed in late convalescence and for the maintenance of joint mobility.

STRENGTHENING EXERCISES

Static or isometric strength can be defined as the maximum force that can be exerted against an immovable object. Dynamic or isotonic strength is a measure of the heaviest weight that can be lifted by concentric (shortening) contractions or lowered by eccentric (lengthening) contractions. Isokinetic dynamic strength is a function of the maximal torque developed at a prescribed rate. In an isokinetic exercise the stress (torque) is kept constant by automatic adjustment of the load (force) as its distance from the joint (fulcrum) changes through a range of movement. Both the rapidity of muscle shortening and the extent of the shortening adversely affect the maximum tension which can be developed.[160, 161]

In general a muscle's strength can be roughly correlated with its bulk or cross-sectional diameter. Within the limitations of the types of strengthening exercises possible in experimental animals, it has been variously shown that strength can increase both with and without evidence of gross muscle hypertrophy.[101, 162, 163] The consensus of most recent studies indicates that high resistance exercise (weight lifting) stimulates white fiber hypertrophy and increases muscle bulk while low resistance, repetitive endurance exercises (distance running) does not significantly increase muscle bulk.[101, 162, 164, 165]

An important consideration in evaluating muscle strength is the method by which strength is measured. The manual muscle test gives a rough approximation of muscle strength useful in the clinical detection of gross evidence of muscular weakness, particularly where a neuropathic or myopathic etiology of weakness is sought.[166-168] The "break test" method advocated by Hines is particularly suitable for bedside detection of gross levels (0 to 4) of muscle weakness.[167] It has been shown by precise measures that strength tested isometrically, regardless of whether a muscle has been trained for strength isometrically or isotonically, will be approximately 13 per cent higher than in the same muscle tested isotonically.[165, 169]

Perhaps of greater interest than strength differences attributable to testing methodologies are the observations that a muscle strengthened by a specific technique, utilizing either a specific movement against resistance (isotonic or isokinetic) or a static resistance in a fixed position (isometric), will give a maximum response if tested in the precise condition in which it was trained.[161, 170-173] Liberson's studies on isometric and isotonic training demonstrated that the isometric-trained subjects did show some improvement on both the static strength test and the one repetition maximum dynamic test, but the carry-over between testing situations was modest.[174]

Precise correlations of muscle strength with electromyographic data have proved difficult. However, the use of the electromyograph has been helpful in assessing the role of motor unit recruitment patterns in achieving the synchrony necessary to forceful contractions.[155, 175,176] The application of full strength or power requires coordination, which in turn is dependent on the synchronous recruitment of motor units. That synchrony in turn is dependent on the highest levels of integration in the nervous system.[169] Both proprioception and motivation will influence the outcome of muscle strength testing.[169]

The important points to make are that, although strength is a function of muscle bulk, it is also influenced by training phenomena and sensory inputs, and that strength tends to be maximal when motivation is maximal and when tested under the conditions that existed during training.

ENDURANCE

STRENGTH-ENDURANCE INTERRELATIONSHIPS

It is evident that in order to endure at a task one has to have the strength to accomplish it. Nonetheless, considerable confusion exists from a semantic standpoint as to the exact meaning of endurance and also from a physiological standpoint as to what constitutes endurance. A major component of muscle endurance is the overall endurance of the individual. This is a function, among other things, of his cardiovascular capability, nutrition, and general health as well as his psychological state.[134, 177-180] This section will be limited to a discussion of endurance as it affects muscle function per se.

Static endurance is either the duration that a specified force can be sustained by a muscle or muscle group or the maximum force that can be sustained for a specified time. Basically, then, static endurance is a function of isometric strength, which in turn is a measure of the strength of muscle under anaerobic conditions. If one's purpose is to train a muscle to be able to hold or sustain a weight for a relatively short period of time — seconds to one or two minutes — then isometric strengthening, which stimulates Type II (glycolysis-dependent) fibers to hypertrophy, is the method of choice.[181-185] Isotonic contractions in which muscles are contracted through their ranges of motion and then *held in a sustained contraction isometrically* accomplish essentially the same purpose but, as discussed below, require the subject to have the capability to move his joints efficiently through the requisite range of motion prior to the sustained contraction.

Dynamic endurance is a measure of the duration that a repetitive act can be maintained and is a function of the rate of repetition, the load, and the extent to which the load is moved. Dynamic endurance is related to but must be distinguished from power, which is the rate at which work (force × distance) is performed. As a consequence of a variety of studies in which histochemical, morphological, electrophysical, and physiological phenomena have been intercorrelated, it is now possible to understand more clearly the distinctions between strength, the various kinds of endurance, and the specificity of the training methods used to achieve them.

It has long been appreciated that red meat or muscles rich in oxygen-binding myoglobin are associated with endurance activities.

The red, myoglobin-rich, wing-beating breast muscles of migrating wild fowl can be contrasted to the white breast meat of the domestic fowl (whose wings beat to facilitate the short hop to a perch). The latter have muscle fibers low in myoglobin and rich in glycogen, as is characteristic for muscles whose actions create high tension of short duration.[186]

The training effect on legs of treadmill running or bicycling or on the arms of rowing has been shown in man to develop predominance of the low-tension, slow-fatiguing, high-oxidative-capacity fibers.[155, 187] The evidence that there is an actual increase in the number of "red fibers" with dynamic endurance training is still being challenged, and the relationships of the fast-twitch and slow-twitch red fibers to power and endurance, as discussed below, are not yet fully delineated.[155, 187-189]

Biochemical, Electrophysiological, and Morphological Correlations

Support has been rapidly accumulating for the characterization of muscle fibers into red (myoglobin-rich) and white, and further distinguishing them as white fast-twitch glycolytic, red fast-twitch glycolytic-oxidative, and red slow-twich oxydative types.[18, 51, 90, 163] The white fast-twitch fibers are associated with high-tension, high-threshold, easily fatigued motor units, and the slow-twitch red fibers are associated with low-threshold, low-tension, fatigue-resistant motor units.[171, 181-185, 190]

Studies on animals in which a weight-lifting exercise was imposed by having them carry a load on their backs while reaching or climbing for food and drink, or in which the load on selected muscles was increased by severing the tendons of their synergists, have demonstrated correlations between muscle strength, hypertrophy, electrical responsiveness, and concentration and characterization of muscle proteins and enzymes.[164, 183-185] Specific histochemical techniques have demonstrated patterns of white fast-twitch fibers, which utilize primarily anaerobic glycolytic metabolic pathways, increased in size and number with static high-resistance stress training, whereas high-oxidative, enzyme-containing slow-twitch fibers increased after low-resistance repetitive (treadmill) activities.[187, 191-193]

This work has been correlated and extended in man by Gollnick and his co-workers, utilizing a needle muscle biopsy technique to study the effect of exercise on both untrained and specifically trained individuals.[187, 191-193] Succinic dehydrogenase activity (oxidative capacity) was found to be much higher in the legs than in the arms of bicyclists, higher in the arms than in the legs of canoeists, and higher in the legs of runners and swimmers than in those of weight lifters (whose succinic dehydrogenase activity generally was no higher than in untrained subjects).[193]

The issues that remain unresolved in this discussion are the relationship of brief isometric contractions to strength and endurance. What is clear from the classic work of Hettinger and Müller is that brief submaximal to maximal isometric contractions of from one to ten seconds' duration once daily are a sufficient physiological stimulus to increase *static* strength without inducing marked fatigue.[174, 194, 195] Further, if the resisted force is progressively increased proportional to the gains in strength, the rate of increase in strength is maximized.[173] Although it is well established that the greater the resisted static force, the more rapid the strengthening effect, a source of confusion is the relationship of this strength, achieved by such a brief effort, to endurance.[173]

To achieve dynamic endurance at a given task one has to have a sufficient minimum of strength to carry out the task and a sufficient reserve to repeat the task at specified intervals. It has been shown in studies of paced, repetitive, isometric hand gripping that even at exercise levels as low as 5 per cent of maximal static hand-grip strength fatigue will eventually occur, and that above 20 per cent of maximal strength fatigue in this exercise is quickly apparent.[196, 197]

Although it has been shown that the ability of an individual to *sustain his maximum grasp contraction* is not directly related to his *maximal grip strength, the ability to sustain a specified low-grade contraction force is a function of the per cent of static strength employed by the muscles involved.* Thus, if one can do a given task using less than 20 per cent of the maximum static strength capability of the muscles employed, the task can be performed efficiently and with less fatigue. In this connection it is of interest that in subjects trained to exhaustion on a bicycle ergometer, stressed at 75 to 90 per cent of maximum voluntary contraction capability, the ability to maintain contractions below 25 per cent of the maximum voluntary contraction force was attributable primarily to the slow-twitch fibers, while above that level it was dependent upon fast-twitch fibers.[193]

MUSCLE-STRENGTHENING METHODS

If a muscle is stressed to the point of fatigue, a "training" effect will occur. This will be manifested by an increase in strength or endurance or both, according to the nature of the stress imposed.[170, 178] Application of this principle has been refined and utilized in gymnastic and therapeutic muscle-strengthening and conditioning exercises. The highly motivating techniques outlined by DeLorme, who prescribed a stepwise reduction of isotonic stress from an initial ten repetitions of a maximal isotonic effort (progressive resistance exercises), and of Hellebrandt, whose "overload principle" involves increasing to the point of fatigue the rate at which a maximum resistance can be overcome, have had wide acceptance.[170, 178, 198]

Another approach which has proved equally successful in increasing strength is the use of brief isometric contractions. The classic work of Hettinger and Müller has shown that brief submaximal contractions can produce a predictable increase in strength without inducing fatigue.[165]

The minimum physiological stimulus to strengthen a muscle requires that a stress of 30 per cent of maximum or greater for the specific muscle be resisted during a contraction of at least one-second duration, once daily.[165] This work is consistent with studies indicating that exercise carried out at various loads greater than 30 per cent of the subject's maximum capability will achieve the same physiological level of strengthening, provided it is carried to the point of fatigue.[170, 178, 199]

Müller more recently has challenged the effectiveness of the 30 per cent maximum contraction as a stimulus and supports work indicating that a two-thirds maximal contraction held for at least one second, and preferably for six seconds, once daily, is the optimal and, in fact, maximal physiological stimulus for isometric muscle strengthening.[173] Extending the duration of the contraction beyond six seconds once daily added very little additional gain in the rate of increase in strength, although a slight increment was observed when the exercise was repeated three times daily.[173] It should be emphasized that the amount of stress must be increased as the muscle strength increases in response to the exercise in order to maintain the rate of increase in strength. Once maximum isometric strength is achieved, it can be maintained by one exercise session per week.[74, 95, 96, 173]

IMPLICATIONS IN ARTHRITIS THERAPY

Muscle weakness and atrophy as a result of pain inhibition or immobility occurs rapidly (at about 30 per cent per week) and therefore, in arthritis and related musculoskeletal disorders, the loss of muscle strength and function for those muscles associated with an arthritic joint is a regularly occurring phenomenon.[194] Smooth coordination of muscle action depends upon sensation, proprioception, and intact central nervous system functioning, but it also requires sufficient strength to carry out the task in a controlled manner.[169] When muscles are weakened as a result of arthritis, the affected joints may be subject to additional stresses as a consequence of the inability of the weakened muscles to provide sufficient synchrony of motion and "shock-absorbing" function.

It has been shown that repetitive joint motion aggravates joint inflammation and that in the presence of intra-articular disease stretching of the joint capsule not only induces pain but inhibits normal muscle function.[133, 139-141] Forceful muscular contractions increase intra-articular pressures and repeated forceful contractions have been associated with increased juxta-articular bone destruction in rheumatoid arthritis.[200, 201] *Strengthening exercises that demand repetitive joint motion or require moving a joint through its range of motion are likely to increase inflammation and pain* in the joint and because of the pain *are unlikely to produce a sufficiently forceful contraction to increase muscle strength.*

Muscle strength sufficient to give static protection to the arthritic joint is a reasonable goal for strengthening exercises. Since a muscle that is taxed at below 20 per cent of its capability can function with relatively little fatigue (and therefore efficiently protect its joint) even on repeated isometric contractions, it is reasonable and possible to design exercises to provide the maximum strengthening effect in a manner that will cause the least possible stress to the arthritic joint.[172, 196]

It has been shown that isometric exercises can strengthen weak muscles acting on an arthritic joint.[174, 202, 203] *The brief maximal isometric contraction performed in an optimal position of comfort* for the patient, such that the force of the contraction will approach maximal (by minimizing pain inhibition), is therefore *the exercise of choice.* This exercise will achieve static strength such that a package can be lifted, steps can be taken, or a patient can change positions from sitting or standing, but it will not of itself permit rapid repeated (dynamic) activities such as walking long distances or prolonged maintenance of posture through repeated minor muscle adjustments.

Carryover from static strength conditioning to dynamic endurance capability is minimal, yet for the arthritis patient the need for dynamic endurance may be a secondary objective.[173] *When sufficient static strength has been achieved* and *when relief of pain is sufficient that repetitive exercises can be tolerated,* then dynamic exercise such as bicycling, swimming, sawing, or weaving can be recommended in order to produce a physiological stimulus for general conditioning, to enhance dynamic endurance in specific muscle groups, and to improve the psychosocial and functional capabilities of the arthritis sufferer.[204, 205]

STRENGTHENING EXERCISES IN MUSCLE DISEASE

Two studies of muscular dystrophy have provided conflicting data on the efficacy of using active isotonic strengthening regimens.[206, 207] Although no apparent ill effects were observed in these studies, it seems reasonable to avoid stressing muscles in the presence of an active myositis or in drug-induced myopathies until sufficient data can be obtained to assess their efficacy. Therefore it is recommended that patients with polymyositis be encouraged to participate in activities as tolerated and not be placed on formal muscle-strengthening regimens until their serum enzymes have returned to normal or at least stabilized. Further, the exercise regimen should be monitored by muscle enzyme determinations to minimize risk of exacerbation of myositis.

SIMPLE TECHNIQUES FOR STRENGTHENING MUSCLES

Although in the therapeutic gymnasium one can utilize strain gauges and weight and pulley systems and special tables to design appropriate isometric or modified isotonic exercise regimens, a simplified technique for isometric strengthening has wider potential applications. This method utilizes an elastic belt so positioned that either one extremity or a fixed object (mattress frame or doorknob) stabilizes the belt and the extremity to be exercised exerts a maximal isometric effort against the resistance of the belt. (See Figs. 45, 46, 48 to 50.) An alternative method is the use of any convenient resistance, such as a tabletop, floor, or the subject's hand (Fig. 43). In the author's experience a partially inflated beachball, which like the belt is lightweight and provides a comfortable surface against which resistance can be applied, offers additionally a sense of resisted tension during compression that provides a proprioceptive stimulus to increase muscle contraction efforts. (See Fig. 44.)

As in stretching exercises, the *daily strengthening-exercise regimen should be performed when stiffness is at its lowest ebb,* when analgesic medication is optimally effective, after hot or cold compresses or a warm shower, or both (but not so long as to be enervating), and with care to place extremities and *joints exercised in a position of maximum comfort.* Assistance may be needed initially during exercise instructions but *active* resistance is essential to increase strength. Significant exacerbation of pain during exercise or lasting more than two hours following exercise or persisting for 24 hours indicates that the exercise program is too strenuous.

EXERCISE TECHNIQUES – APPLICATIONS IN ARTHRITIS

A specific exercise for each of the wide variety of problems encountered in the various joints afflicted by arthritic disorders is beyond the scope of this chapter. Key exercises dealing with common problems in rheumatologic practice — joint mobility or weakness — are selected for emphasis or illustration. References to practical exercise regimens for most arthritic disorders are provided in the subsequent discussions.

THERAPEUTIC EXERCISES FOR ARTHRITIS

ACUTE – SEVERE JOINT DISEASE

Goal: Maintain range of motion (ROM) or minimize loss of ROM and deformity.

Method: Passive or gentle active-assisted ROM.

Position: To avoid gravitational stress and maximize comfort.

Preparations: Cold/heat ± hydrotherapy, analgesia.

Timing: After rest and when stiffness is minimal.

Repetitions: Stretch one to three ROM/session. One to two sessions/day.

Strengthening: Defer until pain permits (see subacute).

Precautions: Range of motion only to point of pain tolerated. Do not cause increased pain or swelling.

Comment: Use resting splints and place extremity in position of function. (See Table 3–1.) A patient with acute and generalized arthritis should be placed in the prone position for 2 hours, total, per day to prevent hip flexion contractures. Teach joint protection and use adaptive equipment to permit function and minimize joint stress in less actively involved joints.

TABLE 3–1. Functional Positions for Ankylosed Joints

Joints	Function	Position	Reference
FINGERS, MCP & PIP	For grasp	35° flexion	282
THUMB, IP	For pinch	Straight	282
MCP	For pinch	20° flexion	
CMC	For apposition	50° abduction	
		20° internal rotation	
WRIST, UNILATERAL		Straight	282
BILATERAL	For ease in toileting	One straight	
		One in 5° flexion	
ELBOW, UNILATERAL	For feeding & grooming	70° flexion	281
BILATERAL	For feeding & grooming	One in 70° flexion	
	For reaching	One in 150° extension	
SHOULDER	For feeding & grooming	20° flexion	280
		45° abduction	
	For dressing	20° internal rotation	
HIP*	For smooth gait	25° flexion	282
		5° abduction	
		5° external rotation	
KNEE**	For smooth gait	15° flexion	284
	10° plantar flexion for high heels	Neutral	284

*Opposite hip, knees, back sitting, walking and other ADL problems must be evaluated to determine the best position.

**Full extension for stability in the knee is the goal when only limited motion can be preserved.

SUBACUTE – MODERATELY ACTIVE JOINT DISEASE

Goal: Maintain or increase mobility and strength.

Method: Active-assisted ROM, isometrics, use of simple exercise equipment.

Position: To avoid gravitational stress and maximize comfort.

Preparations: Heat/cold modality, analgesics prior to therapy as needed.

Timing: When rested and when stiffness is minimal.

Repetitions: Stretch: Three to ten ROM/session. One to two sessions/day. Strengthening: One 6-second isometric/muscle group. One to two sessions/day.

Precautions: An increase of pain lasting over 2 hours or an aggravation of joint symptoms 24 hours after an exercise (or activity) or marked fatigue indicates a need to reduce intensity of the regimen. Do not attempt to stretch without assessing possible structural causes for limitation of passive ROM, including swelling, subluxation, tendon constriction, or nodule impingement.

Comment: Compromises are inevitable between minimizing joint stress and maximizing a meaningful life style. Caution patient against excessive exercise. Use prone position for prophylactic hip flexor stretch. Avoid fatigue. Utilize working splints during activity — dynamic splints are usually not tolerated in the presence of appreciable inflammation. (See Figs. 52 to 56.) Where many joints are affected a practical selection of problem joints for the major focus of exercise therapy may be necessary to obtain adequate compliance, e.g., shoulders, fingers, and knees. Swimming in warm water is the best-tolerated exercise for all-around conditioning.

CHRONIC – MINIMALLY ACTIVE JOINT DISEASE

Goal: Maintain or increase mobility and strength.

Method: Active or active-assisted to stretch; isometric and repetitive isotonic for dynamic strength and endurance. Use of simple exercise equipment.

Position: Comfort. Antigravity exercises when tolerated.

Preparation: Heat/cold modality, analgesia as needed.

Timing: When rested and when stiffness is minimal.

Repetitions: Stretching: Five to ten stretches/session. One session/day to maintain ROM, three to five sessions/day to increase ROM. Strengthening: One 6-second isometric/muscle group/*week* to *maintain* optimal strength.[173] One 6-second isometric/muscle group/*day* to *increase* strength. One set of repetitions of isotonic exercises/day, gradually increasing number of repetitions to tolerance (add one to five repetitions/session) and perform the maximum attained number of repetitions three times/week to maintain dynamic endurance.[211]

Precautions: Same as for Subacute — Moderately Active.

Comments: 1. When only a few joints are involved and the disease activity is minimal, after achieving and maintaining optimal function no further exercise or therapy may be needed. Periodic (4 to 12 month) assessments to assure that function is preserved must then be carried out.

2. Joint contractures (particularly knee) may respond to stretching, but joint dislocations or instability must be supported by increasing muscle strength, stabilizing splints, braces, or surgery.

3. In acute or subacute exacerbations superimposed on chronic joint disease, exercise should be carefully limited to avoid causing a tendon rupture.

4. Generalized chronic active arthritis requires daily maintenance ROM and strengthening exercises in addition to postural, joint protection, and energy conservation measures. In addition, other specific therapy such as splinting and local steroid injections to problem joints is often required. Swimming in warm water is the best-tolerated exercise for all-around conditioning.

EXERCISES FOR SPECIFIC JOINTS

Hand deformities, in fact, all arthritic deformities, are the result of selective involvement of the joint or joints by the disease process, the use and misuse of the joints during activity and rest, and, most important, the persistence and aggressiveness of the disease process in the joint and periarticular involvement.[132] In the rheumatoid hand the metacarpophalangeal (MCP) joint is particularly susceptible to inflammation and the consequent stretching of its capsules and tightening and weakening of the intrinsic muscles. Tenosynovitis in adjacent tendons, articular subluxations, joint destruction or ankylosis in conjunction with variable derangements of proximal interphalangeal (PIP), carpal-metacarpal (CMC), carpal and even distal interphalangeal (DIP) joints lead to the ultimate patterns of deformity.[132]

THE HAND

Common joint problems affecting the hand include restriction of MCP flexion and extension. Restriction of MCP extension is often associated with MCP subluxation, and both MCP flexion and extension are often limited by intra-articular swelling. *Tight intrinsic muscles* (as a consequence of inhibition of painful MCP motion) limit MCP extension and may cause PIP hyperextension (swan neck deformity). (See Fig. 1.) Swan neck deformity can also be caused by a ruptured extensor tendon or a ruptured flexor sublimis tendon.[132] Restriction in passive PIP flexion which is exaggerated when the MCP joints are passively extended (+ Bunnell sign of "intrinsic plus") is attributable to tight intrinsic musculature and is the basis for *intrinsic stretching exercises* designed to minimize MCP subluxation and swan neck deformity. (See Fig. 6.) *Manually assisted* ROM to MCP and IP joints or *exercises utilizing a wooden block* (Bunnell) as a fulcrum for active and active-assisted stretching are used for both articular and intrinsic muscle stretching (Figs. 2 to 6).

Intrinsic and *extrinsic musculature* is usually strengthened by the normally increased hand activities accompanying reduction of pain or by successful therapy for a primary neuromyopathic process (carpal tunnel release). Strengthening by forceful grasping (ball squeezing) activity in the rheumatoid hand predisposes to joint derangement as a consequence of excessive stresses from torques exerted by the flexor tendons on the inflamed MCP joints.[132] If intrinsic muscles are to be put on a strengthening regimen, one six-second isometric exercise of the interosseous and thenar muscles per day performed with the fingers partially extended in a comfortable, painfree position utilizing (1) *manual resistance* from the opposing hand or alternatively (2) *a rubber band* around adjacent fingertips for dorsal interosseous and/or thumb abductor–opponens resistance and (3) *a sponge between* adjacent fingers for volar interosseous or thumb adductor–short flexor resistance should provide the minimal optimal stress.[157, 212-214]

Thumb deformities are a result of the severity and sequence of MCP, IP, and CMC joint and associated tendon involvements.[132] Range of motion exercises to maintain mobility are best performed as two to three stretches, two to three times/day with the manual assistance of the opposite hand. (See Figs. 2 to 4.) Similarly, an effort to maintain mobility in the boutonnière deformity of the PIP joint of the fingers is performed with manual assistance or with pressure on a table top, deck of cards, or "Bunnell block." (See Figs. 5 and 6.)

THE WRIST

Erosion and destruction of the carpi and ulnar styloids are early and characteristic features of rheumatoid arthritis, and the tendency to fusion of the carpi in rheumatoid arthritis, and particularly in juvenile rheumatoid arthritis, is well recognized. Dorsal dislocation of the distal ulnar head, tendon ruptures, carpal tunnel syndrome, and subluxations of the carpi are all frequently observed. The aggravating effect of radial carpal rotations on ulnar deviation of the fingers is well documented.[132, 215, 216] Unfortunately, none of these problems can be prevented by exercise and, in fact, stressful activity of the wrist may predispose to more severe articular and soft tissue damage.

The *objectives of exercise for the wrist* are to *preserve mobility, prevent deformity,* and *maintain strength.* Early involvement of the ulnar aspect of the wrist in rheumatoid arthritis leads to a loss of supination, while radiocarpal and intercarpal swelling and destruction restrict flexion, extension, and, ultimately, pronation as well as radial and ulnar deviation.[157, 212, 217]

Active, and assisted by the opposite hand, daily range of motion exercises for the wrist should include stretching into extension, flexion, ulnar and radial deviation, and pronation and supination. Key exercises include: (1) wrist dorsiflexion (extension) *stretch:* Lean forward with palm placed on a tabletop; perform this exercise two to four times and repeat two to four times daily depending on the severity of inflammation and pain. (See Fig. 9.) (2) *Isometric strengthening* of wrist extensors: Place unaffected hand over dorsum of hand of "affected wrist." Resist maximum extension of wrist for 6 seconds; perform b.i.d. (Avoid in the presence of tenosynovitis of wrist and finger extensors.) (See Fig. 43.) This exercise may be of value in aiding recovery from lateral epicondylitis. (3) *Pronation-supination* stretching using *a lightweight rod as an assisting device:* Elbow at side (placed against lateral chest wall), twist rod outward as far as possible and then inward. Repeat five to ten times, two to four times daily, depending on severity of arthritic involvement and tolerance. (See Fig. 11.)

THE ELBOW

Early loss of elbow extension is a common, although generally not disabling, problem for patients with rheumatoid arthritis. The slight restriction of reach that usually occurs poses no problem, but occasionally there is a marked restriction of elbow extension bilaterally and, more importantly from a functional standpoint, a loss of flexion, pronation, and supination. When loss of elbow flexion is bilateral, eating, for example, is impossible without assistance.

Loss of elbow motion, particularly extension, is difficult to restore, and *attempts to forcefully or vigorously stretch the elbow* into extension *usually only aggravate the problem.*

Elbow extension and flexion range of motion exercises are readily performed with the arm supported on a tabletop. (See Fig. 10.) Repeat exercise five to ten times, two to four times daily, depending on severity and tolerance. Isometric strengthening of elbow flexors and extensors is done with either manual resistance, or the use of a beach ball or an elastic belt.[142, 209, 212] (See Figs. 44 and 45.)

THE SHOULDER

Loss of shoulder (glenohumeral) mobility can be a rapidly occurring process, with significant contracture formation developing within a few weeks. *Aggressive exercise* therapy to overcome contractures before they are irreversible *may necessitate supplementary anti-inflammatory medication* or *local steroid injections* in order to get sufficient pain relief to permit effective exercise.

In cases of severe shoulder pain with marked limitations of motion, as soon as pain tolerance permits, passive (assisted) range of motion exercises to tolerance are supplemented by gravity-assisted *pendulum exercises* (Codman). (See Fig. 12.) These are performed with the patient standing and dangling the arm or lying prone with the affected arm hanging over the side of a bed or treatment table. The addition of a 1- to 2-pound sandbag held in the hand provides additional weight for slight traction and facilitates the pendulum and rotary motions in flexion-extension and circumduction. Two sessions daily with three to ten swings of the arm in flexion-extension and circumduction will help maintain mobility or gently increase motion until about 90 degrees of flexion and abduction is reached.

Exercises to stretch the shoulder beyond 90 degrees progress first to the use of a *reciprocal pulley.* (See Fig. 13.) The unaffected arm pulls down on one end of a rope suspended overhead through a pulley and gently stretches the contractured shoulder into flexion, abduction, or external rotation, depending on positioning. Two to three sessions of five to ten stretches daily are usually well tolerated and effective at this stage. Note: shoulder flexion and abduction are usually lost and restored equally when measured *passively,* but *active* abduction is often more painful than flexion and hence slower to recover. Because active abduction is painful, this exercise should be avoided until late in the restorative program and then performed with the hand supinated in order to avoid painful impingement of the greater tuberosity of the humerus on the coracoacromial ligament.

Somewhat more vigorous than the reciprocal pulley stretching exercise is *"wall walking."* (See Fig. 14.) The patient uses his fingers for support against a wall and "walks" the fingers upward until the arm attains its maximum reach. Flexion, abduction, extension, and internal and external rotation are performed in turn by changing body alignment and proximity to the wall. Marks placed on the wall at the points of maximum stretch create motivating "benchmarks" of progress. The number and frequency of stretches are similar to those used with reciprocal pulleys.

To help restore maximum mobility in the late convalescent phase of a shoulder problem, *batons,* yardsticks, canes, broomsticks, "wands," and the like may be prescribed to assist stretching. These are held in both hands with the "good" arm assisting the affected shoulder in more vigorous stretching through various planes of motion by appropriate movement and positioning of the baton. (See Figs. 15 and 16.) The baton can be moved behind the back for internal and external rotation and can be positioned vertically on the floor behind the head of the bed so that a patient in bed can slide his hand up or down the rod to stretch (10 to 20 stretches in each plane of motion every two to three hours).

Rhythmic stabilization is an effective technique for passive mobilization of the glenohumeral joint, particularly when pain is mild but sufficient to inhibit movement. With the forearm positioned at the extreme of its comfortable range (e.g., abduction-external rotation), a series of alternating strong isometric contractions of abductors and external rotators followed by adductors and internal rotators are made. (See Fig. 17.) Each contraction lasts about 3 seconds, and after two or three cycles of alternating contractions there is usually sufficient muscle relaxation to permit passive motion beyond the previous limit. The whole process is repeated until the maximum range for the session is reached. It can be repeated to supplement other shoulder-mobilizing exercises daily or even weekly until a plateau of maximum range of motion is reached.

Isometric strengthening exercises for the shoulder musculature (6 seconds twice daily) can be easily designed, using a webbed belt or beach ball in a position of comfort, to strengthen the shoulder abductors and external and internal rotators.[142, 158, 212, 217, 218] (See Figs. 44 and 46.)

THE HIP

Hip joint disease leads to a loss in all planes of hip motion, with the loss of extension and abduction and the associated weakness of hip abductors and extensors contributing disproportionately to the loss of function because of their adverse effects on gait and self-care. Maintenance of hip extension by *prone positioning* for 30 to 45 minutes twice daily is a key prophylactic therapy for any patient who is largely confined to bed, regardless of cause, and particularly for patients with neuromuscular disorders or inflammatory hip joint disease. When hip pain is intense, stretching exercises are best done in a *pool*, using water buoyancy to assist in range of motion in extension, flexion, abduction, and internal and external rotation. Stretching in all of these planes of motion can be performed on a *properly positioned*, firm, smooth 1.0 × 1.0 meter *board* (or card table top) *covered with powder* to reduce friction, or with the foot resting in a foot support ("skate") designed to roll easily on casters on the board, tabletop, or floor. Prolonged passive stretching of the hip flexors can be performed with the patient *supine,* a pillow placed so as to raise the affected buttock slightly, and a 10 to 20 lb. weight supported by a sling from the knee. (See Fig. 24.)

Key hip exercises to maintain ROM are performed as follows: (1) (See Fig. 23.) Supine with legs extended, bring knee to chest. Grasp front of knee with hands and pull to chest, keeping opposite leg extended on mat or floor. Repeat five to ten times, alternate legs. (2) (See Fig. 20.) Move extended leg away from midline (abduct) as far as possible. Return to midline. Repeat five to ten times. (3) Feet 10 inches apart, legs extended. Rotate foot outward as far as possible and then inward and repeat five to ten times. Figure 21 illustrates a more vigorous hip rotation exercise. (4) (See Fig. 22.) From a prone position, raise extended leg as high off the mat or floor as possible. Repeat five to ten times. These exercises are performed two to four times daily, depending on the severity of the arthritis and the patient's tolerance.

Isometric strengthening exercises using an elastic belt can be readily performed at home, with particular emphasis placed on strengthening the hip extensor and abductor groups (6 seconds, twice daily).[208, 212, 219] (See Figs. 48 and 49.) The belt can be looped about the knees or ankles in the position of comfort for this exercise so that the maximum resistance can be applied during the contractions.

THE KNEE

Quadriceps weakness is an early and extremely important consequence of arthritis in the knee joint. During ambulation the knee is mechanically stable only in full extension. Contractures of the knee joint capsule and of the hamstring muscles occur as a result of restriction of knee motion due to knee pain and swelling, or secondary to hip flexion contractures. If full knee extension is not possible, stability during ambulation depends largely on the strength of a quadriceps that is invariably weakened from knee arthritis. This predisposes the arthritic joint to increased mechanical stresses and further joint dysfunction.

Knee Range of Motion Exercises. The patient is supine with legs straight; he is instructed to bring his knee to his chest and then grasp his knee with his hands and flex the knee maximally. He returns to the starting position, straightening his leg as fully as possible. Repeat this exercise five to ten times, two to four times daily, as tolerated. Alternatively, perform in a seated position with pulley-assisted knee extension. (See Figs. 25 and 27.)

Isometric Quadriceps Strengthening. The knee position is in slight to moderate flexion to minimize pain. Utilize an elastic belt looped over the ankles for resistance and hold a maximum contraction for 6 seconds, twice daily. (See Figs. 49 and 50.) If pain is fairly acute, exercise for stretching the knee into extension and flexion can be performed in a side-lying position or in a pool in order to relieve gravitational stress. *Deep knee bends should not be done, and bicycling is best avoided until all signs of inflammation have subsided.*[142, 208, 212, 217, 219-221]

THE ANKLE AND FOOT

Persistent inflammation of the ankle leads to restriction of motion and Achilles tendon shortening. Weight-bearing stresses superimposed on the ankle and inflamed proximal tarsal joints result in pronation of the rheumatoid foot and associated peroneal muscle shortening.

Exercises to maintain mobility in the ankle and foot basically involve active or assisted stretching into the normal planes of motion, e.g., ankle: dorsiflexion-plantar flexion; tarsals: foot circling into inversion and eversion; and toes: flexion and extension.

Ankle Range of Motion Exercises.   Position: supine, leg straight, feet relaxed. Point toes toward head, point toes away from head, return to starting position. Turn feet in so that soles are facing each other, curl toes. Turn feet out and straighten toes. Have the patient repeat five to ten times, two to four times each day, depending on the severity of the arthritic involvement and patient tolerance.

Achilles tendon contractures can be prevented by range of motion exercises, but *require vigorous stretching methods,* such as standing on wedged blocks or leaning into a wall and extending the affected leg while holding the heel to the floor for correction. (See Fig. 29.)

Isometric *strengthening* exercises for the *extrinsic foot muscles* are easily performed by pushing or pulling the foot against a beach ball or loop of an elastic belt for 6 seconds twice daily.[142, 212, 219, 220, 222]

Metatarsal-phalangeal joint inflammation leads to intrinsic musculature contractures in the foot. In contrast to the hand, this causes hyperextension of the MTP joints and flexion of the PIPs as well as hallux valgus. The result is painful pressure areas over PIP joints dorsally from shoe (toe box) pressure, and pain on the plantar surface, from walking on the unprotected, depressed metatarsal heads.

Manually assisted mobilization of the toes is used when inflammation is acute. *Active flexion and extension of the toes* for more chronic cases is readily taught by instructing a patient to put one end of a towel on the floor under his feet and draw the rest to him by using his toes like fingers.

THE NECK

The most common cervical problems are associated with discogenic and degenerative disease. Mechanical restriction of lateral flexion and rotation insofar as it is a consequence of lower cervical osteoarthritic bony proliferation will not be affected by efforts to mobilize the neck, but the often large component of restriction of motion that is a consequence of muscle and ligamentous shortening can be effectively stretched. *Neck stretching is best performed with the neck muscles as relaxed* as possible. Pain-induced muscle contractions ("spasms") prevent stretching unless pain can be relieved by a therapeutic modality or medication. Patients often fail in their attempts to deliberately stretch the neck laterally or in rotation. An effective technique for neck stretching has the patient "drop" his head passively so that the chin approaches the chest, then "roll" one ear to a shoulder. The occiput then rolls toward the back, while the chin is rolling to the opposite shoulder and back again to the chest. Repeat twice and reverse. (See Fig. 30.) This should be done with the whole neck and torso as relaxed as possible. It is best done standing, but the patient should be cautioned that it can cause vertigo. This can be tried in rheumatoid arthritis or ankylosing spondylitis but should not be done in the presence of cervical subluxations or radiculopathy.

Rhythmic stabilization exercises are useful in *acute torticollis* as well as in *more chronic painful cervical conditions* where movement of tense muscles increases pain and restricts motion.[117-119] The patient's head is supported and gently turned toward the painful side as far as is comfortably tolerated. The therapist's hands support both sides of the patient's head. The patient is asked to contract the muscles on the painful side by attempting to push the head against the therapist's hand as forcefully as possible. This isometric contraction is held for 2 or 3 seconds and then relaxed. During relaxation the head is laterally rotated or flexed further, as permitted by muscle relaxation, and after a rest of a few seconds the process is repeated. This is continued until maximum stretching has occurred. The whole process is then done in the opposite direction with the goal of inhibiting painful restrictive muscle contraction and restoring full range of motion. This can be repeated daily or twice daily, and some patients with recurring problems can be taught to use this technique independently in a manner similar to manually resisted cervical isometric exercises.

Cervical isometric exercises can be used to preserve or restore musculature weakened by chronic neck pain and *in all patients who wear a brace or collar, as soon as they can be comfortably performed.* (See Fig. 47.) Manual resistance with palm pressure exerted for 6 seconds against the forehead, the occiput and each temple in turn makes a simple once- or twice-daily exercise regimen.[157]

For patients with ankylosing spondylitis, where neck flexion contractures can create a significant handicap, the following neck extension exercise is recommended, unless hip or knee involvement precludes knee flexion exercising. The patient is instructed to stand with his back flat against a wall, to pull his chin in, and then to slide his back up and down the wall by partially flexing and then extending both knees, all the while attempting to hold the back of the head against or as close as possible to the wall. Repeat five times twice daily, increasing to 20 times twice daily.

THE THORACIC OUTLET (SCAPULO-COSTAL) SYNDROME

Weak posterior scapular stabilization and consequent scapular abduction and depression create traction on the levator scapulae, upper trapezii and rhomboid muscles, and this may be associated with pain or contribute to the genesis of the thoracic outlet syndrome (brachial plexus or axillary vessel compression).[223-227]

Postural cues to correct "round shoulders" and to remind patients *to avoid sleeping or working with their arms elevated overhead* and *exercises to stretch tight pectoral muscles* and *strengthen posterior and superior scapular stabilizers* can help relieve symptoms.[227]

Six-second *isometric shoulder "shrugs"* and *scapular abduction exercises are done twice daily.* The patient is instructed to attempt to bring shoulders as close to ears as possible, to hold as forcibly as possible for 6 seconds and then to relax. He then squeezes his shoulder blades as close together as possible, holds them as firmly as possible for 6 seconds, and then relaxes. Vertical "push-ups" are performed with the patient standing and facing a corner with both arms extended horizontally and each palm placed against a separate wall. The patient flexes his elbows and leans toward the corner until his body axis is as far anterior to the elbows as is possible. He then pushes away from the wall and repeats the exercise five to 10 times per session in two to three sessions per day. (See Fig. 19.)

A simpler but less vigorous pectoral stretch can be achieved by clasping both hands behind the neck with the elbows alongside the head and then separating the elbows by externally rotating the shoulders as far as possible. (See Fig. 18.) This exercise should be repeated five to ten times per session as above.[158, 212, 220, 227]

THE DORSAL SPINE AND SPINE EXTENSION EXERCISES

Flexion deformity of the spine is seen by the rheumatologist most often in ankylosing spondylitis, and in osteoporosis with anterior vertebral compression or collapse. *Maintenance of posture is the key objective of therapy* and is aided by the use of a very firm mattress, no pillow, prone positioning with sand bags or bolsters under the chest or thighs (or both) for 30- to 60-minute stretches (while reading, or watching TV) as well as by extension stretching and strengthening exercises.

Exercises to Increase Spine Extension. (1) *Dorsal extension:* The patient is in a prone position, pillow under hips, arms at side, with chin tucked in (to prevent neck hyperextension and strain). (See Fig. 34.) The chest is then raised as far above the mat as possible. Arms are then extended posteriorly as the patient stretches. He then raises both legs and holds for 6 seconds; repeat twice daily. (2) *Lumbar extension:* The patient is prone, with arms at his side. He raises one leg with the knee flexed as far as possible, holds, and returns. This is repeated with the opposite leg until each side is exercised three times. (See Fig. 22.) Both legs are then raised (extended) as high as possible, held for 6 seconds, and lowered. This exercise is done twice each day.

THE LUMBAR SPINE

Exercises for the lumbar spine are designed to relieve low back pain and restore back mobility and function. For the patient with subsiding low back pain, exercises designed to stretch the lumbar and gluteal fascia and muscles (knee-chest and pelvic "tilting") are often helpful in relieving pain.[228, 229] (See Figs. 25, 35, and 36.) Whether any exercise is crucial to the ultimate outcome of lumbar discogenic disease is arguable, but there is good evidence to suggest that abdominal isometric exercises performed so as to minimize intradiscal pressure will assist the recovery of patients suffering from low back pain associated with disc disease. Abdominal muscle strengthening is also beneficial in maintaining muscle tone in those patients who wear a corset or brace.[100, 112, 228, 230-233] (See Fig. 37.)

Quadriceps strengthening by partial or full deep knee bends, if there is no knee problem, is useful to prepare the patient for habitual bending from the knees to spare the back.[100, 228] (See Figs. 38 and 39.) *Pelvic rotation* exercises performed late in the convalescent stage are useful as a relaxing and pain-relieving stretch and as preparation for more vigorous activity. (See Fig. 21.)

Progressive Exercises for Subsiding Acute Low Back Pain. Each exercise is added in turn only when it is established that the preceding exercise is well tolerated. All exercises should be performed deliberately and under full control.

(1) *Circulation exercise:* For patients on bed rest. Plantar-flex and dorsiflex ankles ten times each hour when awake (to minimize venous clot formation).

(2) *Pelvic tilt:* (See Fig. 35.) To stretch lumbar fascia and strengthen glutei.[228, 234] The patient lies supine with the knees bent and feet flat. Both hands are placed on the upper abdomen to help limit movement to the lumbosacral region. While keeping the back flat on a mat or the floor, the pelvis is rotated away from the mat by contracting pelvic and gluteal muscles. The movement is repeated three to five times as a stretch and held for 6 seconds on the final "tilt" as an isometric strengthening contraction. This exercise usually increases the patient's comfort and should be repeated three to five times per day.

(3) *Knee chest:* (See Figs. 25 and 36.) To stretch lumbar and gluteal muscles.[228, 234] The patient lies supine with knees flexed and feet flat. One knee is flexed to approach the axilla and returned. This is repeated on the opposite side, alternating from side to side for five repetitions. If pain permits, it should be performed bilaterally after the initial alternating stretch is completed, as that permits a greater stretch. Return one leg at a time to starting position to avoid uncontrolled movement. This is repeated five times, three to five times per day.

(4) *Abdominal isometric strengthening:* (See Fig. 37.) The patient is

supine with knees flexed, feet flat, and back flat. The neck is flexed.[234] The arms are extended with the fingers reaching to or over but not touching the knees. The upper back should be raised off the floor or mat. This is held for 6 seconds and repeated twice daily. The patient is instructed to exhale, or count out each second, or say "Mississippi" slowly two times to prevent a Valsalva effect. When this can be done easily, to maximize the strengthening effect the contraction should be held until fatigue occurs.

(5) *Deep knee bends with wall support:* To increase quadriceps and gluteal strength and endurance, and to reinforce use of squatting rather than bending forward to pick up objects. The patient stands with his back flat against a wall and his heels 4 inches away from the wall.[228, 234] He is instructed to slide down the wall, keeping his back flat by bending his knees until a semi-sitting position is reached, and then return to standing by sliding back up the wall. Initially this is done five times, three times each day. If there is no knee problem and this exercise is easily done, proceed to deep knee bends. If there is a knee problem or if deep knee bends are too difficult, continue with a similar sequence of partial to full deep knee bends but without wall support, using a chair back or tabletop for balance. (See Figs. 38 and 39.)

(6) *Knee bends without wall support:* The patient stands facing the back of a chair or tabletop and places one or both hands on the chair back (or tabletop) for balance. He tilts his pelvis, keeping his spine flat, and bends his knees as previously described. This again commences with five knee bends, three times per day, and is increased gradually to 30 knee bends, three times per day.

(7) *Pelvic rotation:* (See Fig. 21.) The patient is supine with knees bent and feet flat. He places the right foot on top of the left knee and slowly attempts to lower the left knee (right foot is overlapping left knee), assisted by the right foot to the floor or mat. The shoulders are kept flat during the exercise. He returns to the starting position and reverses the exercise, lowering the right knee to the floor. Both rotations are repeated five times, twice daily. This exercise is also useful for stretching tight hip external rotators. None of these exercises should cause any discomfort other than what one would expect from gentle stretching.

SELECTED READINGS BY TOPICS

(See also complete Bibliography on page 213.)

Rest and Relaxation

108. Gault, S. J., Spyker, M. J.: Beneficial effect of immobilization of joints in rheumatoid and related arthritides: a splint study using sequential analysis. Arthritis Rheum., *12*:34, Feb. 1969.

113. Watkins, R. A., Robinson, D.: *Joint Preservation Techniques for Patients with Rheumatoid Arthritis.* Chicago: Northwestern University, 1974. P. 16.

Stretching Exercises

125. Cooke, A. F., Dowson, D., Wright, V.: Lubrication of synovial membrane. Ann. Rheum. Dis., *35*:56–59, Feb. 1976.
135. Harris, E. D., Jr., Evanson, J. M., DiBona, D. R., et al.: Collagenase and rheumatoid arthritis. Arthritis Rheum., *13*:83, Jan.–Feb. 1970.
140. Agudelo, C. A., Schumacher, H. R., Phelps, P.: Effect of exercise on urate crystal–induced inflammation in canine joints. Arthritis Rheum., *15*:609, Nov.–Dec. 1972.
142. Preston, R. L.: *The Surgical Management of Rheumatoid Arthritis.* Philadelphia: W. B. Saunders Co., 1968. Pp. 77, 203, 214–219, 288.
143. American Rheumatism Association, Arthritis and Rheumatism Foundation and National Institute of Arthritis and Metabolic Diseases: *Chapter 3. Evaluation of Splinting.* Criteria for the evaluation of orthopedic measures in the management of deformities of rheumatoid arthritis. Arthritis Rheum., 7(5):Part 2:585, 1964.
144. Stein, H., Dickson, R. A.: Reversed dynamic slings for knee-flexion contractures in the hemophiliac. J. Bone Joint Surg., *57A*:282, Mar. 1975.
150. Flatt, A. E.: "Chapter 3. Nonoperative treatment," *in* A. E. Flatt, ed., *The Care of the Rheumatoid Hand.* 3rd Ed. St. Louis: C. V. Mosby Co., 1974. P. 33.
151. Bunnell, S.: *Surgery of the Hand.* 5th Ed. Revised by J. H. Boyes. Philadelphia: J. B. Lippincott Co., 1970. P. 297.
152. Fried, D. M.: "Chapter 13. Splints for arthritis," *in* S. Licht, ed., *Arthritis and Physical Medicine.* Baltimore: Waverly Press, 1969.
209. Swezey, R. L: Exercises with a beach ball for increasing range of joint motion. Arch. Phys. Med., *48*:253, May 1967.

Strengthening Exercises

155. Edington, D. W., Edgerton, V. R.: *The Biology of Physical Activity.* Boston: Houghton Mifflin Company, 1976. Pp. 55, 280.
157. Kendall, P. H.: "Chapter 26. Exercise for arthritis," *in* S. Licht, ed., Therapeutic Exercise. 2nd Ed. New Haven: E. Licht, 1965. P. 707.
158. Cailliet, R.: *Shoulder Pain.* Philadelphia: F. A. Davis Company, 1966. P. 45.
165. Hettinger, T.: Physiology of Strength. Edited by Thrulwell, M. H. Springfield, Illinois: Charles C Thomas, 1961.
166. Hines, T. F.: "Chapter 8. Manual muscle examination." *in* S. Licht, ed., *Therapeutic Exercise.* New Haven: E. Licht, 1965. Pp. 175, 163.
167. Daniels, L., Worthingham, C. A.: *Muscle Testing: Techniques of Manual Examination.* 3rd Ed. Philadelphia: W. B. Saunders Co., 1972. P. 16.
170. DeLateur, B. J., Lehmann, J. F., Fordyce, W. E.: A test of the DeLorme axiom. Arch. Phys. Med. Rehabil., *49*:245, May 1968.
173. Müller, E. A.: Influence of training and of inactivity on muscle strength. Arch. Phys. Med., *51*:449, Aug. 1970.
187. Gollnick, P. D., Armstrong, R. B., Saltin, B., et al.: Effect of training on enzyme activity and fiber composition of human skeletal muscle. J. Appl. Physiol., *34*:107, Jan. 1973.
199. DeLateur, B. J., Lehmann, J. F., Giaconi, R.: Mechanical work and fatigue: their roles in the development of muscle work capacity. Arch. Phys. Med. Rehabil., *57*:319, July 1976.
202. Machover, S., Sapecky, A. J.: Effect of isometric exercise on the quadriceps muscle in patients with rheumatoid arthritis. Arch. Phys. Med. *47*:737, Nov. 1966.
208. Magness, J. L., Lillegard, C. Sorenson, S., et al.: Isometric strengthening of hip muscles using a belt. Arch. Phys. Med. Rehabil., *52*:158, Apr. 1971.
264. Lehmann, J. F., Warren, C. G.: Restraining forces in various designs of knee ankle orthoses: their placement and effect on the anatomical knee joint. Arch. Phys. Med. Rehabil., *57*:430, Sept. 1976.

Exercises for Specific Joints

119. Long, D. M.: Electrical stimulation for relief of pain for chronic nerve injury. J. Neurosurg., *39*:718, 1973.
158. Cailliet, R.: *Shoulder Pain.* Philadelphia: F. A. Davis Company, 1966, P. 45.
212. Toohey, P., Larson, C. W.: *Range of Motion Exercise: Key to Joint Mobility.* Rehabilitation Publication No. 703, Sister Kenny Institute, Minneapolis, Minnesota, 1968. Pp. 2–39.
219. Fried, D. M.: "Chapter 12. Rest versus activity," *in* S. Licht, ed., *Arthritis and Physical Medicine.* Baltimore: Waverly Press, 1969. P. 270.
221. Cailliet, R.: *Knee Pain and Disability.* Philadelphia: F. A. Davis Company, 1973. P. 57.
222. Cailliet, R.: *Foot and Ankle Pain.* Philadelphia: F. A. Davis Company, 1968. Pp. 89–110.
227. Britt, L. P.: Nonoperative treatment of the thoracic outlet syndrome symptoms. Clin. Orthop., *51*:45, Mar.–Apr. 1967.
228. Williams, P. C.: The conservative management of lesions of the lumbo-sacral spine. The American Academy of Orthopaedic Surgeons. Instructional Course Lectures. Michigan: American Academy of Orthopaedic Surgeons. 1953. P. 90.
233. Nachemson, A.: Towards a better understanding of low-back pain: a review of the mechanics of the lumbar disc. Rheum. Rehabil., *14*:129, Aug. 1975.
234. Cailliet, R.: *Low Back Pain Syndrome.* 2nd ed. Philadelphia: F. A. Davis Company, 1965. Pp. 58–70.

A PORTFOLIO OF
ILLUSTRATIONS

STRETCHING EXERCISES*

HAND

1. Intrinsic Muscle Anatomy
2. Manually Assisted DIP Range of Motion
3. Manually Assisted PIP Range of Motion
4. Manually Assisted MCP Range of Motion
5. Bunnell Exercise – DIP Flexion, PIP Extension
6. Bunnell Exercise – DIP and PIP Flexion with Stretch of Intrinsic Musculature
7. PIP Traction-Assisted Stretching
8. MCP Traction-Assisted Stretching

WRIST-ELBOW

9. Wrist Dorsiflexion (Assisted Stretching)
10. Elbow Flexion-Extension (Friction-Assisted [Desk Top] Gravity Eliminated [Horizontal Position])
11. Elbow-Wrist Pronation-Supination (Active, Assisted with a Rod or Lightweight Hammer)

SHOULDER

12. Codman Exercise (Gravity-Assisted)
13. Reciprocal Pulley (Pulley-Assisted)
14. "Wall Walking" (Friction-Assisted [wall])
15. Wand-Assisted Exercise #1
16. Wand-Assisted Exercise #2
17. Rhythmic Stabilization (Manually Assisted Manipulation)

---

*Some strengthening exercises are included here with the stretching exercises because a forceful isometric contracture is readily incorporated at the end of the stretching process.

49

18. Pectoral Stretch (Active)
19. Pectoral Stretch by "Vertical Push-up" (Active Assisted Pectoral Stretch with Terminal Isometric Strengthening of Shoulder Stabilizers)

HIP

20. Hip Abduction-Adduction (Active Stretch of Adductors)
21. Hip-Pelvis Internal Rotation (Active Assisted Stretch of External Rotary Components of Hip and Lumbosacral Fascia)
22. Hip Extension (Active Extension Stretch of Hip and Lumbar Flexor Musculature)
23. Hip Flexion (Active, Manually Assisted Stretch of Hip Extensors During Flexion, with Simultaneous Stretch of the Hip Flexors on the Opposite, Extended Side)
24. Hip Extension (Passive, Weight-Assisted Stretch of Hip Flexors)

KNEE

25. Knee Flexion — Alternating Knee Chest (Manually Assisted Stretch of Knee Extensors and Lumbosacral Fascia)
26. Knee Extension (Passive, Weight-Assisted Stretch of Knee Extensors
27. Knee Flexion-Extension, Seated (Active, Friction-Assisted [floor] Flexion with Passive, Pulley-Assisted Extension)
28. Knee Extension, Traction-Assisted

ANKLE

29. Ankle Dorsiflexion (Active Assisted Gastrocnemius–Soleus–Achilles Tendon Stretch)

NECK

30. Neck Rotation (Active, Gravity-Assisted)
31. Cervical Traction

BACK — ANKYLOSING SPONDYLITIS

32. Kneeling-Rocking (Shoulder-Spine-Hip Flexion-Extension)
33. Crawling in Place (Shoulder-Spine-Hip Flexion-Extension)
34. Upper Spine Extension (Active Stretch of Spine Flexors)

LOW BACK—LUMBOSACRAL EXERCISES

35. Pelvic Tilt (Active Stretch of Lumbar Fascia, with Terminal Isometric Hold for Gluteal Strengthening)
36. Bilateral Knee-Chest (Active Stretch of the Lumbar and Gluteal Fascia)
37. Abdominal Isometric Exercise (Strengthening of Abdominal Musculature)
38. Partial Deep Knee Bend (Dynamic Endurance Exercise for the Quadriceps and Gluteal Muscles)
39. Deep Knee Bends (Dynamic Endurance Exercise for Quadriceps and Gluteal Muscles) (See Illustration #38)
40. Side Lying or "Hook" Lying Position (Initial Step in Transferring from Lying to Standing Position)
41. Semi-seated Supported Position (Step 2 in Transferring from Lying to Standing)
42. Seated, Manually Supported Position (Step 3 in Transfer Process)

STRENGTHENING EXERCISES

43. Wrist Extensor Strengthening (Manually Resisted Isometric Contraction of Wrist Extensor)
44. Biceps Strengthening (Beach Ball–Resisted Isometric)
45. Biceps-Triceps Strengthening (Belt–Resisted Isometric)
46. Shoulder, Deltoid–External Rotator Strengthening (Belt-Resisted Isometric)
47. Neck Flexor Strengthening (Manually Resisted Isometric)
48. Hip Abductor Strengthening (Belt-Resisted Isometric)
49. Quadriceps and Opposite Gluteal-Hamstring Strengthening (Belt-Resisted Isometric)
50. Quadriceps Strengthening (Seated, Belt-Resisted Isometric)

POSTURE, SPLINTS, AND BRACES

51. Posture, Sitting
52. Static Wrist Stabilizing (Working) Splint
53. Ulnar Deviation Splint
54. Thumb IP Stabilizing Splint
55. Thumb CMC-MCP Stabilizing Splint—Plastic
56. Thumb CMC-MCP Stabilizing Splint—Leather
57. Trigger Finger, PIP Splint—Elastic
58. Below Knee Weight-Bearing (BKWB) Brace
59. Oxford Shoe with SACH Heel and Rocker Sole
60. Shoe-Heel Lift (Leg Length) Correction (A & B)
61. Philadelphia Cervical Brace

ASSISTIVE DEVICES

STRETCHING EXERCISES

HAND

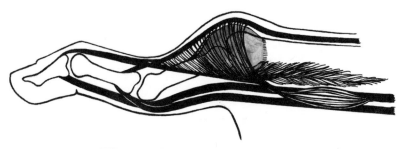

FIGURE 1. Intrinsic muscle anatomy

Contractures of the interosseous and lumbrical muscles as a consequence of meta-carpophalangeal (MCP) joint inflammation create tension on the finger extensor tendon mechanism. The result is MCP flexion and proximal interphalangeal (PIP) hyperextension. Elasticity of the large flexor digitorum profundus muscle creates traction on the distal interphalangeal (DIP) joint. The result is a swan neck deformity. **See pages 23 and 35.**

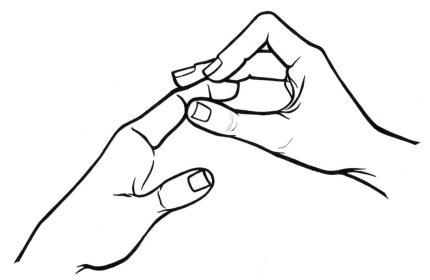

FIGURE 2. MANUALLY ASSISTED DIP RANGE OF MOTION (STRETCHING)

Flexion and extension of the DIP joint is assisted by the opposite hand. **See Cases 8 and 17. See pages 25 and 36.**

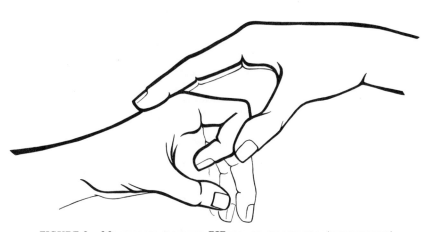

FIGURE 3. MANUALLY ASSISTED PIP RANGE OF MOTION (STRETCHING)

Flexion and extension of the PIP joint is assisted by the opposite hand. **See Cases 8 and 17. See pages 25 and 36.**

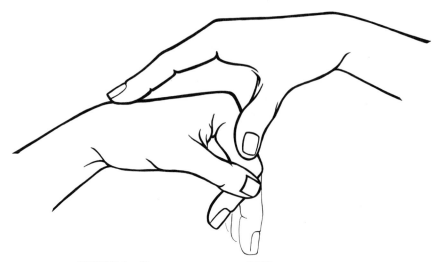

FIGURE 4. MANUALLY ASSISTED MCP RANGE OF MOTION

The MCP joint is flexed and extended with manual assistance of the opposite hand. **See Cases 8 and 17. See pages 25 and 36.**

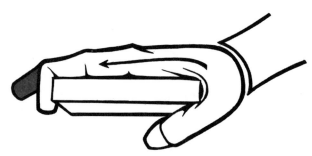

FIGURE 5. BUNNELL EXERCISE – DIP FLEXION, PIP EXTENSION (STRETCHING)

The flexion contracture of the PIP joint is extended against a wooden block or deck of cards. This can be enhanced by manual assistance of the opposite hand. This exercise is useful in extension contractures of the DIP, flexion contractures of the PIP joints and in early boutonnière deformities. **See Cases 8 and 17. See page 36.**

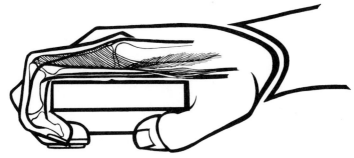

FIGURE 6. **B**UNNELL **E**XERCISE—**DIP** AND **PIP** FLEXION WITH STRETCHING OF
INTRINSIC MUSCULATURE

The lengthening of the long finger extensor tendons that occurs as the fingers are flexed around the block, with the MCP joints kept in extension, stretches the tight intrinsic musculature. This exercise is useful in early swan neck deformities and in metacarpophalangeal flexion contractures. **See Cases 8 and 17. See page 36.**

FIGURE 7. **PIP**–TRACTION-ASSISTED
STRETCHING*

Spring wire "knuckle bender" brace. Rubber bands create tension on a spring wire brace that can be positioned to overcome extension or flexion contractures of the PIP joints. This device, shown here positioned to stretch a flexion contracture, is used after inflammation has largely subsided and is applied for periods varying from 20 minutes to one hour, as tolerated. Rubber band tension is made gentle and the device can usually be tolerated intermittently at 1- to 4-hour intervals throughout the day. Traction is terminated when after two weeks of consistent usage no further change in joint range can be demonstrated. **See Cases 8 and 17. See pages 24 and 112.**

*Although not properly an exercise, this traction-assisted brace is included for convenience here because it represents part of a logical sequence of increasingly more vigorous stretching activities for the hand.

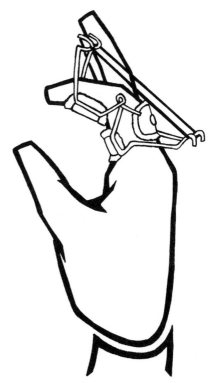

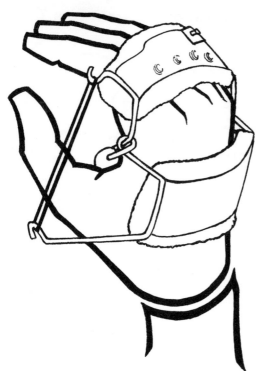

FIGURE 8. MCP–TRACTION-ASSISTED STRETCHING

Spring wire "knuckle bender" brace. Rubber bands create tension on a spring wire brace that is designed to overcome extension contractures of the MCP joints. This device is used after inflammation has largely subsided and is applied for periods varying from 20 minutes to one hour as tolerated. Rubber band tension is made gentle and the device can usually be tolerated intermittently at 1- to 4-hour intervals throughout the day. Traction is terminated when after two weeks of consistent usage no further change in joint range can be demonstrated. **See Cases 8 and 17. See pages 24 and 112.**

WRIST–ELBOW

FIGURE 9. WRIST DORSI-FLEXION (ASSISTED STRETCHING)

The affected hand is placed on a table top and supported by the opposite hand. The body is gently leaned forward, creating leverage to stretch a contracture on the volar aspect of the wrist. **See Case 17. See pages 25 and 37.**

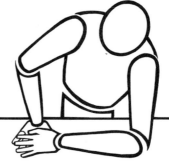

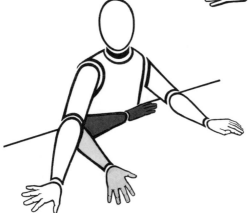

FIGURE 10. ELBOW FLEXION-EXTENSION STRETCHING (FRICTION-ASSISTED [DESK TOP] GRAVITY ELIMINATED [HORIZONTAL POSITION])

The forearm is placed on a desk top for support. The elbow is flexed and extended, utilizing the support of the table as well as the friction of the table to assist in stretching. **See Case 6. See pages 25 and 37.**

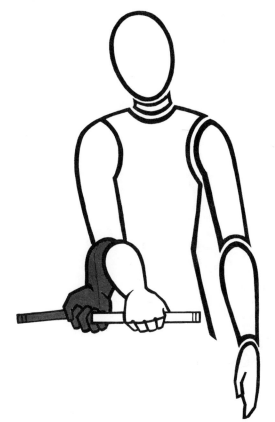

FIGURE 11. Elbow-wrist
pronation-supination
stretching (active-assisted
with a stick or light-
weight hammer)

The wrist and elbow are
pronated and supinated as the
stick is rotated. Shoulder motion
is eliminated by the position of
the forearm adjacent to the chest
wall. **See Case 6. See page 37.**

SHOULDER

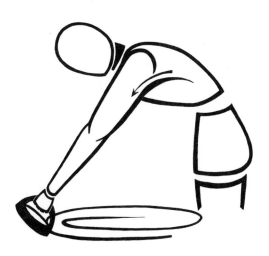

FIGURE 12. Codman
exercise (gravity-assisted
stretching)

The patient bends forward
and gravity assists the shoulder
and arm in a rotary and/or pendulum motion to stretch into
flexion, extension, and abduction.
This can be performed with a
patient standing or lying prone
over the edge of a bed. In the
standing position the exercise is
best performed with the patient
supporting himself by leaning on
a table top or chair. **See Cases 5
and 17. See pages 25 and 38.**

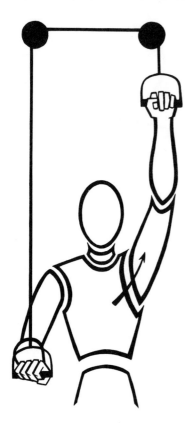

FIGURE 13. RECIPROCAL PULLEY
(PULLEY-ASSISTED STRETCHING)

The "good" arm pulls down on one end of the pulley system and assists the affected arm in stretching. Changing the patient's position under the pulley system permits assisted stretching in the various planes of motion. **See Cases 5 and 17. See pages 25 and 39.**

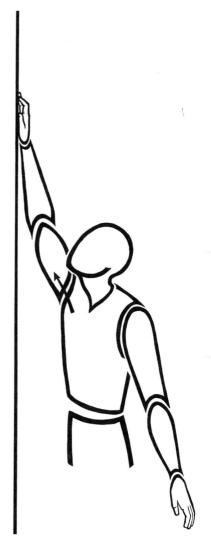

FIGURE 14. "WALL WALKING"
(FRICTION-ASSISTED [WALL] STRETCHING)

Friction between the fingers and the wall assists in actively stretching the shoulder. A mark placed at the highest attained stretch provides a guide to progress. Flexion and abduction are effectively stretched by facing the wall and standing parallel to it respectively. **See Cases 5, 16, 17. See page 38.**

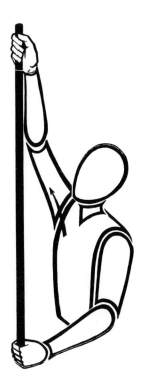

FIGURE 15. WAND-ASSISTED EXERCISE #1
(STRETCHING)

A stick, cane, baton, or wand is held in the unaffected hand, which assists ranging of the affected shoulder by pushing or pulling in the desired direction. Forward flexion is illustrated above. With the wand placed behind the back, external rotation or internal rotation can be performed. This exercise can be employed in the presence of moderately active inflammation of the shoulder and is particularly useful when efforts are being made to restore mobility at a time when inflammation has largely subsided. **See Cases 5, 16, and 17. See pages 35 and 38.**

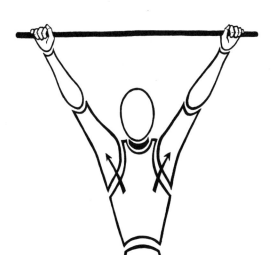

FIGURE 16. WAND-ASSISTED
EXERCISE #2 (STRETCHING)

In this exercise the wand in the unaffected hand assists in a bilateral stretching movement. This exercise is enhanced by visual monitoring when performed in front of a mirror. **See Cases 5, 16, and 17. See page 38.**

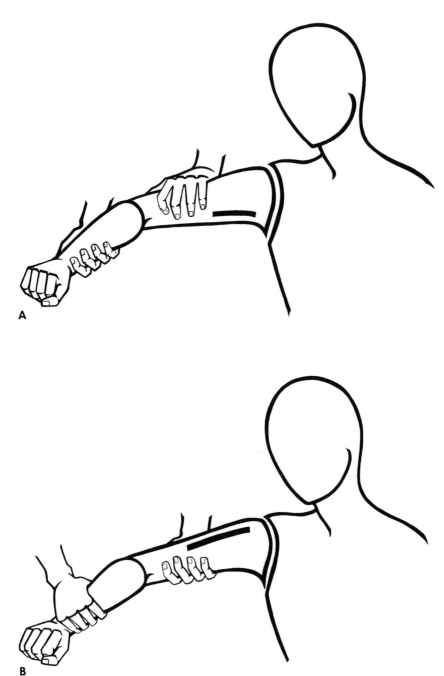

FIGURE 17.   *See legend on opposite page.*

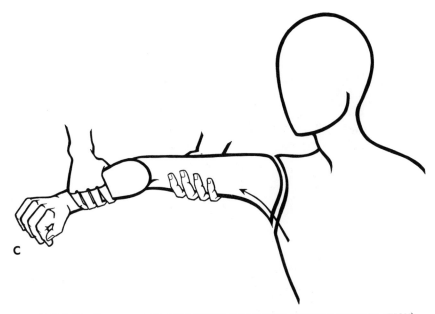

FIGURE 17. RHYTHMIC STABILIZATION (MANUALLY ASSISTED MANIPULATION)

This is basically a passive stretching method, shown here as it is applied to the shoulder. The forearm is positioned in the extreme of its comfortable range and then a series of alternating strong isometric contractions of abductors and/or external rotators followed by adductors and internal rotators are made. Each contraction is held for about three seconds and the series of contractions consists of two or three cycles of alternating agonist and antagonist contractions. The muscle relaxation that follows the period of contractions is usually sufficient to permit the "manipulator" to passively move the joint beyond the previous limit. This process is then repeated until the maximum range for the session is attained. Rhythmic stabilization sessions can be performed daily and used as a supplement to other shoulder-mobilizing exercises, and may be effectively repeated as infrequently as weekly until a plateau of maximum range of motion is achieved. This same method can be employed in patients with painful muscle spasm limiting cervical motion.

In Figure *A* alternating resistance to internal rotation and extension of the shoulder is shown.

In Figure *B* alternating resistance to the external rotators and abductors of the shoulder is shown. In actuality the arm is placed in the position of maximum tolerated external rotation and abduction with resistance initially applied to the internal rotators and/or extensors, as this is the direction of least discomfort. This contraction is then cycled with a contraction in the same position of the external rotators and/or abductors and then alternated again with the internal rotators, as described above.

Figure *C* shows the relaxed shoulder (post-rhythmic stabilization) passively stretched or lifted to the newly tolerated range of motion. **See Case 17. See pages 22 and 39.**

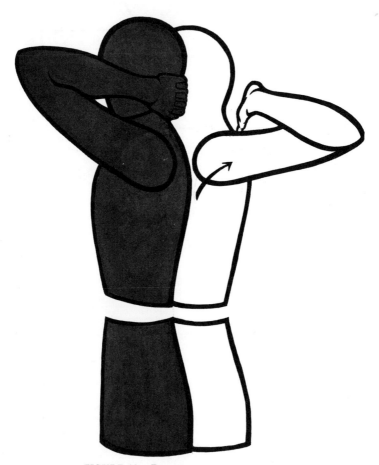

FIGURE 18. PECTORAL STRETCH (ACTIVE)

Both hands are clasped behind the neck with the elbows alongside the head. The elbows are then separated by externally rotating the shoulders as far as possible. This pectoral muscle stretch can be effectively combined with an isometric strengthening contraction of the posterior scapular stabilizers at the end of the stretch. **See Cases 4 and 18. See page 43.**

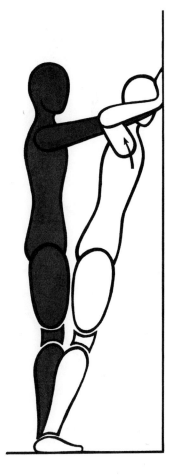

FIGURE 19. PECTORAL STRETCH BY "VERTICAL PUSH-UP" (ACTIVE-ASSISTED PECTORAL STRETCH WITH TERMINAL ISOMETRIC STRENGTHENING OF SHOULDER STABILIZERS)

The patient stands with his arms horizontal to the floor and his hands placed against the wall or on either side of the corners of a wall. He allows his body to lean into the wall as far as possible, while keeping his feet flat. He then pushes away from the wall and repeats this as a series of stretching exercises. An isometric contraction in the inclined position strengthens the shoulder stabilizers. Combining deep breathing with the stretching in Exercises 18 and 19 is particularly useful in patients with restricted chest expansion due to ankylosing spondylitis. **See Cases 4 and 18. See page 43.**

HIP

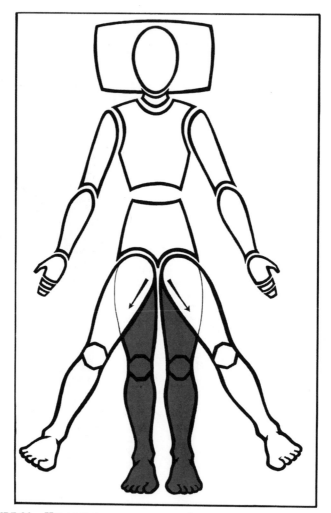

FIGURE 20.   Hip abduction-adduction (active stretch of adductors)

The patient is supine with gravity eliminated. The legs are moved away from the midline and then returned in a series of stretching motions. This can be done alternately on one side and then the other or bilaterally. The use of a smooth gliding surface such as a powder board, or performance of this exercise in water can facilitate the stretching. If performed unilaterally, crossing one leg over the other, the exercise can serve as a hip abductor stretch. **See Case 14. See pages 25 and 39.**

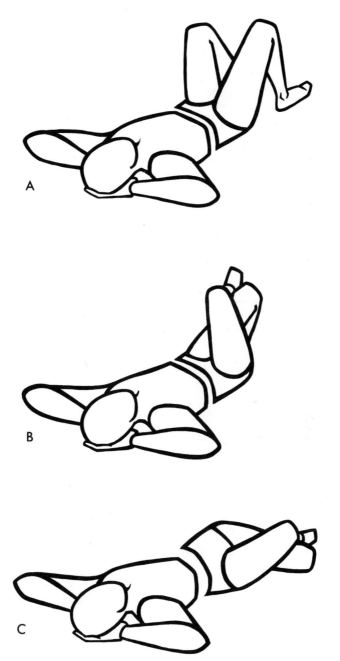

FIGURE 21. HIP-PELVIS INTERNAL ROTATION (ACTIVE-ASSISTED STRETCH OF EXTERNAL ROTARY COMPONENTS OF HIP AND LUMBOSACRAL FASCIA)

The patient is supine with knees flexed and feet flat on the floor. The foot of one leg is placed on the outside of the opposite knee. The foot then helps to push the knee of the internally rotating hip toward the floor. The patient's upper back and shoulders remain in the starting position to permit maximum rotation at the hip and lumbosacral area. **See Cases 13 and 14. See pages 25, 39, 44 and 45.**

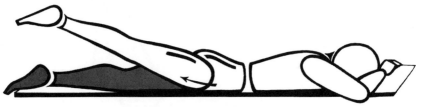

FIGURE 22. HIP EXTENSION (ACTIVE EXTENSION STRETCH OF HIP AND LUMBAR FLEXOR MUSCULATURE)

The patient is prone and alternately raises each leg as high as possible, returning it to the starting position before repeating the procedure on the opposite side. This exercise may be better tolerated if it is initially performed in the side-lying position. An isometric strengthening contraction at the extreme of hip extension can be added, if tolerated, at the end of the series of stretches. **See Cases 4 and 14. See pages 39 and 43.**

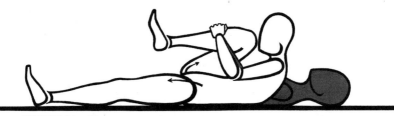

FIGURE 23. HIP FLEXION (ACTIVE, MANUALLY ASSISTED STRETCH OF HIP EXTENSORS DURING FLEXION WITH SIMULTANEOUS STRETCH OF THE HIP FLEXORS ON THE OPPOSITE EXTENDED SIDE)

The patient is supine. While keeping one leg fully extended on the floor or a mat, the opposite leg is flexed and assisted into maximum flexion with the hands placed over the tibia. In some patients this may create stress at the knee joint and the hands are then placed behind the distal femur. Neck and upper spine flexion augment the stretch throughout the entire spine. This exercise is a more vigorous knee flexion, hip flexion, and lumbosacral flexion stretch than that shown in Figure 25. **See Cases 14 and 15. See pages 39 and 43.**

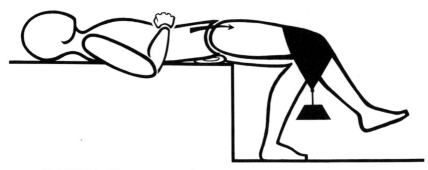

FIGURE 24. HIP EXTENSION (PASSIVE, WEIGHT-ASSISTED STRETCH OF HIP FLEXORS)

This is performed when an early hip flexion contracture is detected. A weight of approximately 10 kilograms is suspended from a sling over the affected hip for periods of 20 to 40 minutes, three to four times daily until the contracture is overcome or stabilized. A small pillow under the pelvis just proximal to the affected hip creates a comfortable fulcrum to enhance stretching. **See pages 24 and 39.**

KNEE

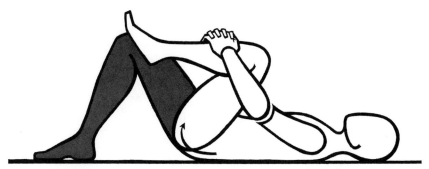

FIGURE 25.   **KNEE FLEXION–ALTERNATING KNEE-CHEST (MANUALLY ASSISTED STRETCH OF KNEE EXTENSORS AND LUMBOSACRAL FASCIA)**

The patient is supine with both knees flexed. Alternately, one knee and then the other is brought to the chest, with flexion manually assisted by grasping the anterior surface of the tibia. This exercise is also a gentle stretch of the lumbosacral fascia and can be used early in the recovery from discogenic disease and lumbosacral strain. **See Cases 11 and 13. See pages 25, 40 and 44.**

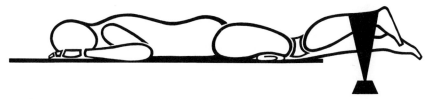

FIGURE 26.   **KNEE EXTENSION (PASSIVE, WEIGHT-ASSISTED STRETCH OF KNEE EXTENSORS)**

The patient is prone, lying obliquely on a bed or treatment table with the affected lower leg off the bed. A 5- to 10-kilogram weight is suspended by a sling from the dorsum of the ankle, and the knee is passively stretched for a period of 20 to 40 minutes. This method is useful in mild chronic knee contractures. The same procedure can be done in a seated patient with the leg supported at the heel on a chair placed in front of the patient. The sling is then suspended over the dorsum of the knee and the weight pulls the knee into extension from below. **See page 24.**

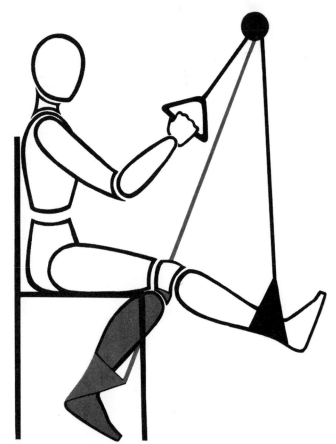

FIGURE 27.   KNEE FLEXION-EXTENSION STRETCHING, SEATED (ACTIVE
FRICTION-ASSISTED [FLOOR] FLEXION WITH PASSIVE PULLEY-ASSISTED EXTENSION)

This exercise is performed when active range of motion causes excessive discomfort. The patient utilizes a pulley to assist in knee extension stretching and slides his foot along the floor to help increase flexion. **See pages 25 and 40.**

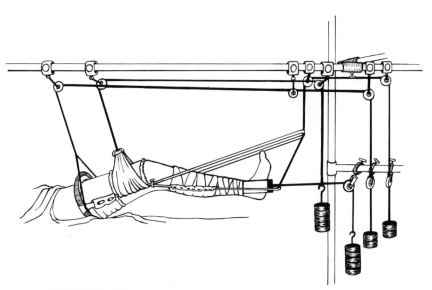

FIGURE 28. KNEE EXTENSION, TRACTION-ASSISTED (STRETCHING)

A modified Russell's traction with a sling suspension placed so that a 3- to 10-kilogram weight transmits (via a pulley system) a downward pressure over the dorsum of the knee. A horizontal distracting force of 3 to 10 kilograms creates a simultaneous distraction of the tibia on the femur. Three-kilogram weights are used to counterbalance the weight of the leg by attachment to the proximal ring and distal stirrup of the reversed Thomas splint. **See pages 24 and 139.**

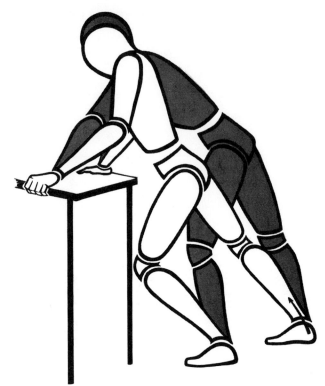

FIGURE 29. ANKLE DORSIFLEXION (ACTIVE-ASSISTED GASTROCNEMIUS–
SOLEUS–ACHILLES TENDON STRETCH)

This is a vigorous stretch of the ankle plantar flexors. The patient stands before a table and extends the affected leg posteriorly. He then flexes the opposite knee while attemping to keep the foot of the affected ankle flat on the ground. By leaning toward the table or bouncing and leaning toward the table, the ankle plantar flexors are stretched. **See page 41.**

NECK

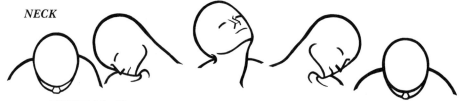

FIGURE 30. NECK ROTATION (ACTIVE, GRAVITY-ASSISTED STRETCHING)

The patient is seated or is standing and supporting himself with his hands on a chair back. He assumes an extremely relaxed posture of his entire body and allows his head to slump forward in a chin-down position. The head is rotated so that the right ear falls toward the right shoulder (ear to shoulder); in this rotated position the neck and upper trunk move into extension as the head rolls or rotates so that the chin slides over to and "falls" on or near the opposite shoulder (chin to shoulder). The head continues to roll forward with the chin approaching the chest and the cycle is repeated twice. The whole process is then reversed. The key to this exercise is relaxation. The positions are not achieved by deliberate placement of the head but rather by a relaxed, rolling movement. It is useful to advise the patient to feel like a "rag doll" in order to emphasize the lack of deliberate forced head positioning which tends to be counterproductive. Although standing allows for freer body movement, light-headedness and actual vertigo can be precipitated by this exercise, and for susceptible patients it is best performed in a sitting position. This exercise is performed twice daily. **See Case 9. See pages 41 and 42.**

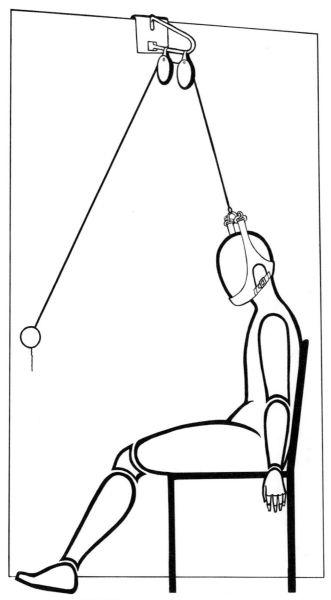

FIGURE 31. CERVICAL TRACTION

A simple over-the-door traction apparatus is utilized. The patient is seated alongside the door in such a manner that when the tractive force is applied his head is in approximately 20° of flexion and centered so that the line of pull of traction does not deviate the head and neck from the midline. The patient, preferably in an armless chair, sits up straight and applies the halter so that when traction is applied, support is equally distributed between the chin and the occiput or is slightly greater at the occiput. He then relaxes his body and slumps in the chair and allows the weight of the upper body to serve as a traction force. This technique eliminates the need for any complex apparatus or struggling with weights. Some patients are not able to relax sufficiently to utilize this method, or the tractive force of their body weight is excessive, in which cases specific weights (7 to 15 kg) are used in the traction pulley system. Where no weight is used the suspending rope can be either tied to the overhead pulley or attached to an adjacent doorknob. **See Cases 9 and 10. See page 139.**

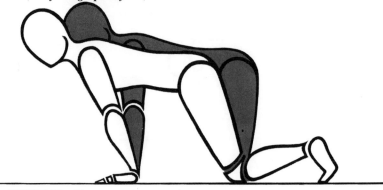

FIGURE 32. KNEELING-ROCKING (SHOULDER SPINE HIP FLEXION-EXTENSION STRETCHING)

The patient kneels on the floor or on a bed and rocks back on his haunches and forward over his hands and alternately places his back in an arched or sway position. This is an excellent "loosening-up" exercise for patients with generalized morning stiffness. **See Case 4. See page 25.**

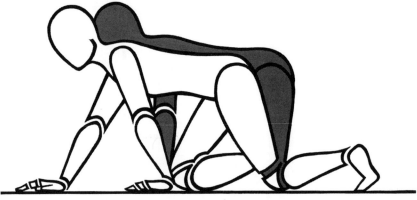

FIGURE 33. CRAWLING IN PLACE (SHOULDER-SPINE-HIP FLEXION-EXTENSION STRETCHING)

This is a second phase of Exercise #32. The patient alternately reaches with an arm and a leg in crawling-in-place motion or actually crawls. This provides a controlled stretch to the shoulders and hips and spine and serves as a mobilizing exercise to relieve morning stiffness and as a prelude to more vigorous exercise therapy. **See page 25.**

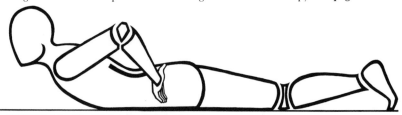

FIGURE 34. UPPER SPINE EXTENSION (ACTIVE STRETCH OF SPINE FLEXORS)

The patient assumes a prone position with arms at sides and attempts to clear the chest from the mattress or floor and then resumes the prone position. At the end of the series of stretches an isometric six-second "hold" serves as an additional muscle-strengthening exercise that supplements the anti-gravity stretch.*

*See Cases 18 and 19 for pectoral stretch and deep breathing. See Figure 22 for hip and low-back extension exercises. See Exercises 38 and 39 for deep knee bends and associated spine postural cues.

LOW BACK (Lumbosacral Stretch)

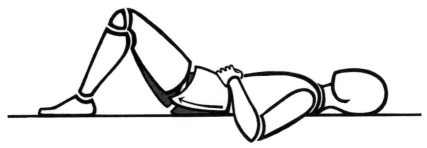

FIGURE 35. **PELVIC TILT (ACTIVE STRETCH OF THE LUMBAR FASCIA, WITH TERMINAL ISOMETRIC HOLD FOR GLUTEAL STRENGTHENING)**

The patient is supine with the lumbar spine flattened against the floor or mat and both knees flexed and feet planted. The hands are placed over the lower abdomen in order to help reinforce the flattened lumbar spine position. The pelvis is tilted posteriorly. (This is perceived as a sensation of the anterior superior iliac spines moving away from the hands placed on the abdomen as well as by a sense of lifting in the sacro-coccygeal region.) The gluteal muscles are tightened during this movement, and a firm isometric contraction at the termination of the full pelvic rotation or pelvic tilt adds an isometric strengthening of the gluteal muscles to the stretch of the lumbosacral fascia. This exercise is useful as an initial exercise in a back reconditioning program because it is usually well tolerated. It also provides a means of creating an awareness of the flattening of the lumbar spine that occurs during posterior tilting of the upper pelvis. It is an effective exercise to relieve discomfort associated with chronic stiffness in the low back or stiffness that is aggravated by poor sleeping or sitting posture. **See Cases 11, 13, and 15. See page 44.**

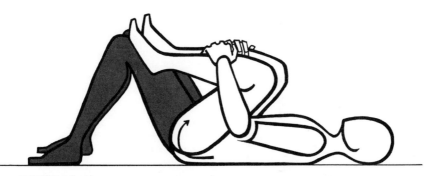

FIGURE 36. **BILATERAL KNEE-CHEST (ACTIVE STRETCH OF THE LUMBAR AND GLUTEAL FASCIA)**

This exercise is usually introduced after the alternating knee-chest exercise shown in Figure 25. The bilateral knee-chest exercise is a somewhat more vigorous stretch of the lumbosacral fascia. Care must be taken that both legs are lowered carefully to the starting position with knees flexed. Initially, this should be done with one leg lowered at a time. **See Cases 11, 13, and 50. See page 44.**

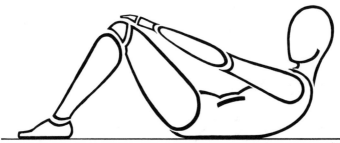

FIGURE 37.   ABDOMINAL ISOMETRIC EXERCISE (STRENGTHENING OF ABDOMINAL MUSCULATURE)

This is exclusively a strengthening exercise but is placed here because it is a key exercise in a back reconditioning program and is usually introduced after pelvic tilt and knee-chest exercises. The patient is supine with the knees flexed and the feet flat. Keeping the lumbar spine flat, he attempts to lift the upper dorsal spine and head so that the hands reach to or over the knees. This position is held initially for a count of six to provide an adequate isometric strengthening stimulus. Ultimately this is increased to a point of fatigue just short of that which would preclude a controlled resumption of the supine position. The patient exhales or counts out loud during the isometric contraction (as in all isometric exercises). **See Cases 11, 13, and 15. See page 44.**

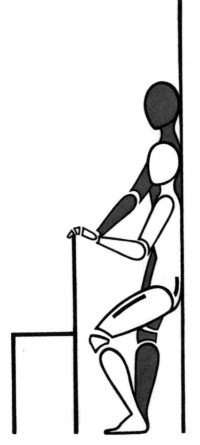

FIGURE 38.   PARTIAL DEEP KNEE BEND (DYNAMIC ENDURANCE EXERCISE FOR THE QUADRICEPS AND GLUTEAL MUSCLES)

This is a dynamic endurance conditioning exercise that is placed here because it is the appropriate next step in a sequence of increasingly more vigorous back reconditioning exercises. The exercise as shown shows the patient utilizing the back of a chair for support. While partially lowering and raising himself, the spine is kept flattened and the movements are controlled. This exercise is best initiated with the patient standing with his back to a wall and his heels three or four inches away from the wall. He then slides up and down utilizing the wall as a support. In this technique he learns to flatten his entire spine against the wall and thereby to reinforce a posture which puts minimal stress on the lumbosacral fascia and underlying structures. The exercise also serves to remind the patient to assume the proper standing posture and use flexion of the knees and hips or a squatting posture to retrieve low-lying articles or fallen objects. The exercise is repeated initially three to five times and progresses until approximately 40 knee bends can be accomplished rhythmically and under control. **See Case 13. See pages 44 and 45.**

FIGURE 39. **Deep knee bends
(dynamic endurance for quadriceps
and gluteal muscles)
(See Figure 38.)**

This is a more vigorous exercise than the preceding one and further helps to prepare patients to retrieve objects from the floor as well as to increase their overall physical fitness. Hip and knee and occasionally ankle problems may preclude the use of the deep knee bend. **See Case 13. See pages 44 and 45.**

Note: See Figure 21. The pelvic rotation exercise shown in Figure 21 can be introduced, if tolerated, following successful accomplishment of the preceding exercises in patients with chronic low back pain and discogenic disease. The pelvic rotation exercise is useful in relieving chronic stiffness in the lumbosacral region and in restoring rotation of the pelvis and the lower lumbar spine.

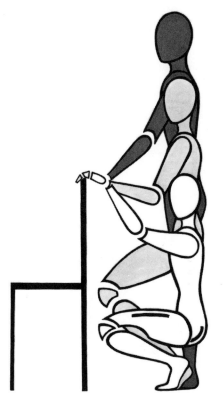

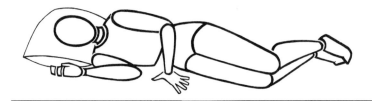

FIGURE 40.   SIDE LYING OR "HOOK" LYING POSITION (INITIAL STEP IN
TRANSFERRING FROM LYING TO STANDING POSITION)

The patient is generally most comfortable in this position with the hips and knees moderately flexed, the lumbar spine flat, and the neck supported. A firm mattress is essential for support during transfer. **See Cases 11, 12, 13, and 15. See pages 101 and 127.**

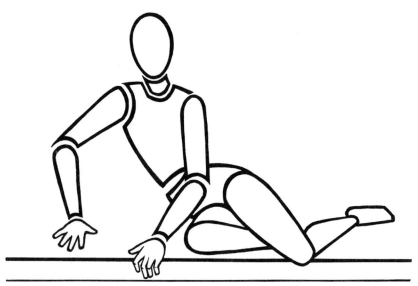

FIGURE 41.   SEMI-SEATED SUPPORTED POSITION (STEP 2 IN
TRANSFERRING FROM LYING TO STANDING)

Using both arms for support, the body is carefully moved into a semi-seated position. The upper pelvis is tilted posteriorly. **See Cases 11, 12, 13, and 15. See pages 101 and 127.**

FIGURE 42. SEATED MANUALLY
SUPPORTED POSITION (STEP 3
IN TRANSFER PROCESS)

With careful arm support the
patient has lowered first one leg
and then the other so that he assumes a sitting position. From this
position the patient keeps his back
firm and slides to the edge of the
bed. He then carefully partially
rotates to one side, sliding his feet
to the floor one at a time, the outer-
most foot first. With one hand supported on the mattress and the
lumbosacral angle kept flat he
rises in a controlled manner to assume the standing posture. The
entire process is reversed in a stepwise fashion on returning to bed.
**See Cases 11, 12, 13, 15. See pages
101 and 127.**

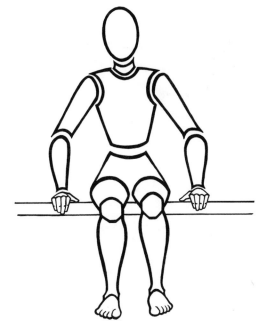

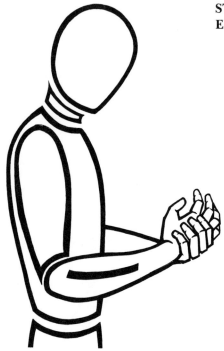

STRENGTHENING EXERCISES*

FIGURE 43. **WRIST EXTENSOR STRENGTHENING (MANUALLY RESISTED ISOMETRIC CONTRACTION OF WRIST EXTENSORS)**

The patient uses one hand placed over the dorsum of the other hand to resist extension during a maximum isometric contraction of six seconds' duration. **See Cases 6 and 17. See pages 32 and 37.**

FIGURE 44. **BICEPS STRENGTHENING (BEACH BALL–RESISTED ISOMETRIC)**

A partially inflated beach ball is forcibly squeezed until no further movement is possible, and the isometric contraction is held for six seconds. The compression of air within the beach ball yields until it offers maximal resistance. The compression gives proprioceptive feedback to reinforce the strength of the muscle contraction. The exercise is performed for six seconds at maximal compression. The beach ball can be placed in various positions to exercise different muscle groups, e.g., between the lateral thigh and a wall for isometric hip abductor strengthening. **See Cases 6 and 17. See pages 32, 37 and 39.**

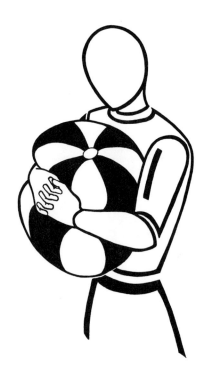

*See Fig. 18, scapular isometric strengthening exercise; Fig. 22, low back isometric exercise; Fig. 24, upper back isometric exercise; Fig. 35, gluteal isometric exercise; and Fig. 37, abdominal isometric strengthening exercise. Exercises 38 and 39 are quadriceps and gluteal dynamic endurance and strengthening and conditioning exercises.

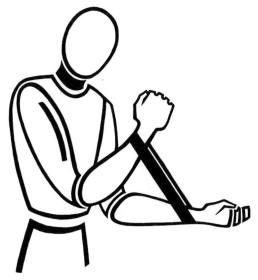

FIGURE 45. BICEPS-TRICEPS STRENGTHENING (BELT-RESISTED ISOMETRIC)

The right biceps and left triceps in this illustration are opposed in an isometric contraction resisted by an elastic band or belt. The elasticity is such that at the maximum contraction no motion is possible and the tension of the elastic band provides proprioceptive stimulation to encourage a maximally forceful contraction for isometric strengthening. The contraction is held for six seconds. **See Cases 6 and 17. See pages 32 and 37.**

FIGURE 46. SHOULDER DELTOID—EXTERNAL ROTATOR STRENGTHENING (BELT-RESISTED ISOMETRIC)

The elastic band or belt is looped over both wrists. Abduction and external rotation of the right shoulder is resisted by the opposite arm. The maximum contraction is held for six seconds and the exercise is performed once or twice daily. **See Cases 5, 16, and 17. See pages 32 and 39.**

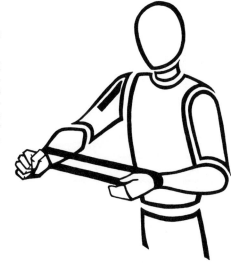

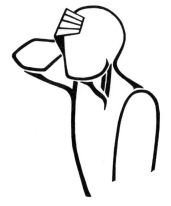

FIGURE 47. NECK FLEXOR STRENGTHENING (MANUALLY RESISTED ISOMETRIC)

The hand is placed on the forehead and resists contraction by the neck flexors. The neck extensors, lateral flexors and rotators can be similarly exercised with the hand placed to offer resistance appropriately. Each contraction is held for six seconds and the exercise is performed once to twice daily. **See Cases 9 and 18. See pages 42 and 122.**

79

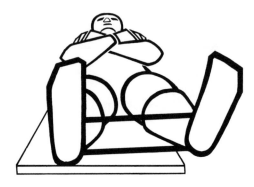

FIGURE 48. Hɪᴘ ᴀʙᴅᴜᴄᴛᴏʀ
STRENGTHENING (BELT-
RESISTED ISOMETRIC)

The belt is looped over both ankles. The left hip abductors attempt a maximum contraction against the resistance of the belt. Strengthening stimuli occur in both the stabilizing extremity and the extremity being "exercised." Where the opposing extremity is too weak to stabilize the contraction an alternative fixation of the belt can be employed, as in Figure 50. **See Case 14. See pages 32 and 40.**

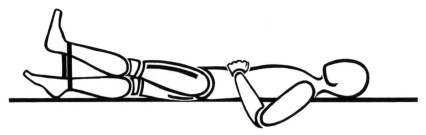

FIGURE 49. Qᴜᴀᴅʀɪᴄᴇᴘs ᴀɴᴅ ᴏᴘᴘᴏsɪᴛᴇ ɢʟᴜᴛᴇᴀʟ-ʜᴀᴍsᴛʀɪɴɢ sᴛʀᴇɴɢᴛʜᴇɴɪɴɢ
(ʙᴇʟᴛ-ʀᴇsɪsᴛᴇᴅ ɪsᴏᴍᴇᴛʀɪᴄ)

An elastic band or belt is looped over both ankles. In this exercise the quadriceps of the left or near leg is strengthened. There are simultaneous isometric contractions of the proximal hip extensors and hamstring musculatures in the stabilizing opposite leg. The isometric contraction is held for six seconds and the exercise is performed once to twice daily. **See Cases 5 and 14. See pages 32 and 40.**

FIGURE 50. **QUADRICEPS STRENGTHENING (SEATED, BELT-RESISTED ISOMETRIC)**

The belt is looped around a leg of the chair for stability and the left leg attempts to overcome the belt resistance by a maximum contraction. In this illustration the knee is placed in mid-range to minimize pain and enhance the possibility of a forceful contraction. In addition to the convenience of exercising in this position, the possibility that the opposite leg is incapable of offering sufficient resistance to the contraction is obviated by the use of the chair for stabilization. The contraction is held for six seconds and the exercise is performed once to twice daily. **See Case 15. See pages 32 and 40.**

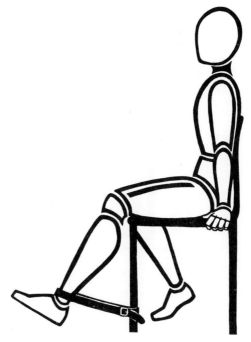

POSTURE, SPLINTS AND BRACES*

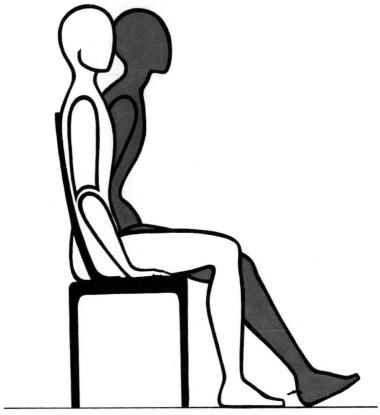

FIGURE 51. Posture, sitting

For proper alignment in the seated posture the placement of the head is such that the external auditory meatus is on a plumb line that extends laterally through the shoulder and the greater trochanter. In a standing posture this line is extended to pass on the anterior lateral surface of the knee and to terminate (with the foot flat on the floor) on a point just anterior to the ankle. When seated the spine should be supported by the back rest, and this is facilitated by allowing ample space for the buttocks to protrude posteriorly or to be supported by an appropriately shaped and cushioned back support. The thighs are horizontal or in approximately 95° of flexion, the knees in 90° of flexion, and the feet are planted (with the ankles at 90°) firmly on the floor or on a stool. There should be approximately the width of a fist between the popliteal space and the sloped and preferably padded surface of the anterior surface of the chair to minimize pressure on popliteal neurovascular structures. There should be room between the chair legs so that the feet can be placed beneath the chair to facilitate transfer to the standing position. Alternatively, one or both feet may be placed on a low stool or on a strut fitted between the rockers of a rocking chair. The exact seating alignment will depend on the activities engaged in while sitting, and they may range from slight reclining for relaxation, television viewing, and relaxed reading to the vertical position, shown above for desk work or eating. The contrasted figure is illustrated in a slumped posture that creates hyperextension and stress on the neck and hyperflexion and stress on the lumbosacral junction. **See Cases 12 and 18. See pages 100 and 128.**

*See Figures 7 and 8.

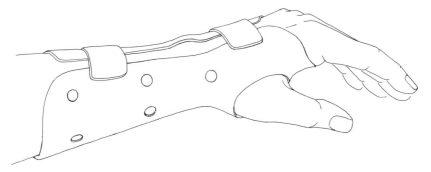

FIGURE 52. STATIC WRIST STABILIZING (WORKING) SPLINT

This splint is a custom-molded thermo-labile plastic splint. It extends from distally just proximal to the distal palmar crease to the proximal one-third of the forearm. There is a wide aperture for thumb clearance. It is useful in arthritis of the wrist and to prevent hyperflexion and hyperextension of the wrist in the carpal tunnel syndrome. **See Cases 1 and 2. See pages 34, 105 and 111.**

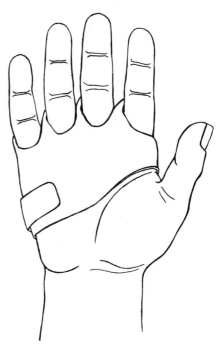

FIGURE 53. ULNAR DEVIATION SPLINT

This is a thermo-labile plastic custom-molded splint that extends from the distal one-third of the proximal phalanges to end just proximal to the distal creases. It is designed to permit only partial MCP flexion but full PIP and DIP motion. A vane on the ulnar side of each finger resists ulnar deviation. The thumb is free; the dorsal strap and Velcro closure hold the splint in place. This splint may improve function in patients with severe ulnar deviation. Its value in prophylaxis or correction of ulnar deviation is not established. **See Case 2. See pages 34 and 111.**

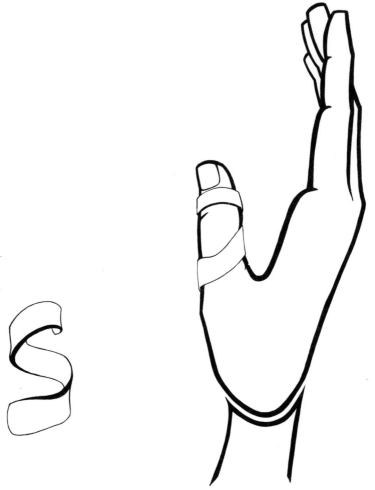

FIGURE 54.   THUMB IP STABILIZING SPLINT

The splint is metal and designed as a coil. The palmar coil lies just proximal to the IP joint, allowing for flexion of that joint, while the two dorsal surfaces of the coil resist IP extension. There is maximal thumb skin surface exposed to facilitate sensation and function. The splint can be fabricated out of plastic but when a thermo-labile plastic material is used it cannot be worn during exposure to warm surfaces or hot water. **See Case 2. See pages 34 and 112.**

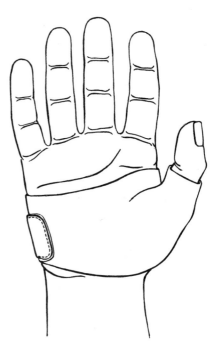

FIGURE 55. THUMB CMC-MCP
STABILIZING SPLINT, PLASTIC

This is a thermo-labile plastic custom-molded splint designed to provide moderate restriction of the CMC and MCP joints of the thumb. It allows for full IP flexion in order to permit optimal thumb function. The distal palmar edge of the splint is proximal to the distal palmar crease so as not to restrict MCP motion in the fingers. This splint is useful in CMC and MCP arthritis of the thumb and in DeQuervain's disease. **See Case 19. See pages 34 and 112.**

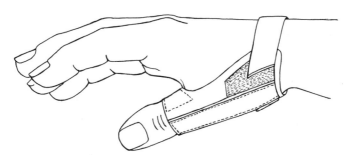

FIGURE 56. THUMB CMC-MCP STABILIZING SPLINT, LEATHER

This is a commercially fabricated splint similar in purpose to that shown in Figure 55. Its advantages are that it does not require a custom fit and if waterproofed it can be used in warm water. The disadvantages are that the long thumb post may obstruct some IP flexion and it may give insufficient support to the thumb. **See pages 34 and 113.**

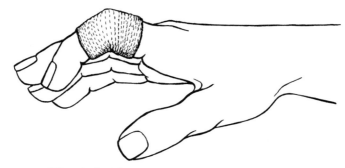

FIGURE 57. Trigger finger PIP splint, elastic

This is a one-inch-wide elastic band sewn to make a snug (not tight) sleeve overlying the PIP joint of a finger. The elasticity permits flexion of the PIP joint from zero (extension) to about 60 to 70° of flexion. This mild restriction of PIP flexion is compatible with most functions but restricts the full excursion of the flexor tendons and thereby minimizes tenosynovial irritation and "triggering." **See Case 20. See page 113.**

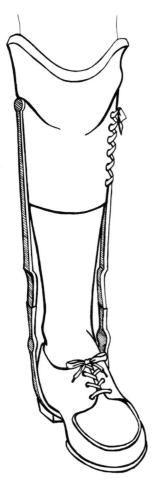

FIGURE 58. Below knee weight-bearing (BKWB) brace

This brace consists of a plastic or leather molded infrapatellar upper calf cuff designed to be closely approximated to the upper one-third to one-half of the calf. A lateral and medial metal strut fixed to the shoe transmits the bulk of the body's load away from the foot and onto the lower calf. When ankle motion is painful the ankle hinge is eliminated. Ankle motion is then simulated by a SACH heel and a rocker sole. (See Figure 59.) This brace is useful in relieving stress on chronic painful refractory ankle, hindfoot and heel conditions. **See Case 3. See page 115.**

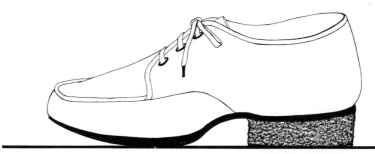

FIGURE 59.   OXFORD SHOE WITH SACH HEEL AND ROCKER SOLE

The SACH, or cushion, heel absorbs the shock at heel strike and is yielding enough to give way sufficiently during the stance phase of gait to allow the foot-flat stage to be reached with only minimal ankle movement. If the cushion heel is too soft it will cause an unsteady stressful gait. The rocker sole is combined with a rigid internal shoe shank to stabilize the tarsal and MTP joints. The foot rolls over the rocker sole into the toe-off phase of gait with minimum motion of these joints or of the ankle. The cushioned heel is useful in some cases of heel pain. The rocker sole is useful in osteoarthritis of the first MTP or IP joint and when combined with a metatarsal pad may relieve the pain of severe MTP arthritis. The combination of a SACH heel and rocker sole is indicated for chronic ankle or hind foot (proximal tarsal) arthritis. Note that a proper shoe for an arthritic foot or ankle should: (1) support the heel with a firm heel counter, (2) support the midfoot with a rigid shank, preferably with multiple lacing, and (3) allow ample room for the toes with a high toe box and a wide anterior (metatarsal area) last. Seams should not be located over dorsally protruding toe deformities. **See Case 3. See page 115.**

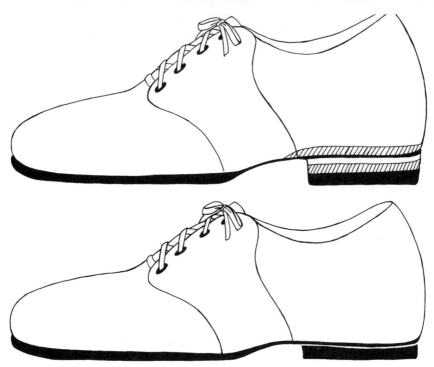

FIGURE 60. SHOE—HEEL LIFT (LEG LENGTH) CORRECTION

A. A ¹/₈ to ¹/₄ inch correction can be applied inside or outside the heel. A combination of ¹/₄ inch inside and ¹/₄ inch outside the heel allows for a ¹/₂ inch correction. This usually does not cause forefoot stress and obviates the necessity to provide additional sole thickness and weight.

B. Removal of ¹/₄ inch from the opposite heel is shown. This combination of ¹/₂ inch added to one shoe and ¹/₄ inch removed from the other shoe permits a total correction of ³/₄ inch with good cosmesis, little added shoe weight, and no stressful foot positioning. **See Case 11. See page 119.**

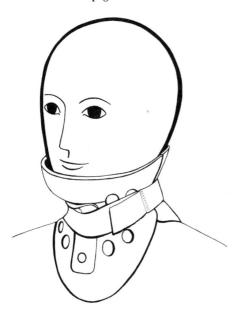

FIGURE 61. PHILADELPHIA CERVICAL BRACE

This is a plastic, commercially available brace which is readily adjusted and comfortable to wear. It provides good stabilization of the entire spine and is especially effective for stabilizing the lower cervical vertebrae. It has occipital, submental, and upper thoracic contact points. It is useful in moderate to severe cervical problems that do not require absolute immobilization. For cervical support in bed it serves as a comfortable alternative to the slightly more efficient but more uncomfortable SOMI brace (Fig. 62). The chief disadvantage of the Philadelphia brace is that it tends to be uncomfortable in warm weather. For most cervical problems in which severe subluxations and/or neurological complications have not occurred, the use of a soft felt or foam rubber padded collar, or a plastic or plastic and metal collar, designed without specific suboccipital, submental, or chest contact points, will usually provide sufficient stabilization to provide pain relief. **See Case 10. See pages 120 and 121.**

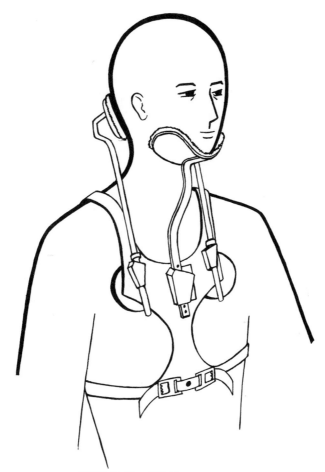

FIGURE 62. **SOMI** CERVICAL BRACE

A plastic and metal rigid brace that requires careful adjustment and fitting. Firm occipital and submental supporting plates are rigidly held by a removable bar to a chest plate. The chest plate is held firmly to the chest by over-the-shoulder and under-the-arm straps. This brace provides excellent stabilization of the lower cervical spine and is comparable to the fourposter or Philadelphia braces in stabilization of the middle and upper cervical areas. It tends to be uncomfortable and is particularly difficult to wear when lying down. It is useful for the patient with mild radicular deficits that do not require absolute cervical stabilization. **See Case 10. See pages 120 and 121.**

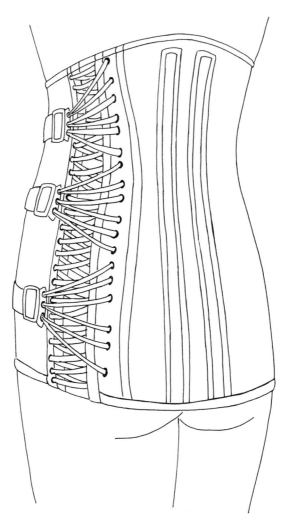

FIGURE 63. Lumbosacral corset or belt

This is a fabric corset that has adjustable lacing for snugness and is reinforced laterally and posteriorly by flexible or rigid stays or both. The "belt" is essentially a "male corset," more rigidly stayed posteriorly and usually designed with lateral lacing. Rigid stays are most efficient in restricting lateral motion but reduce comfort and ease of fitting. This corset should extend just above the lower ribs and anchor beneath the curve of the buttocks. Firm approximation of all surfaces and abdominal compression are essential to the proper fit. Rib compression may be painful and necessitate corset modification. There should be sufficient space so that compression of the upper anterior thigh does not occur when sitting. The lumbosacral corset or belt is indicated for moderate to severe low back pain, with or without radiculopathy. **See Cases 11, 12, and 13. See page 124.**

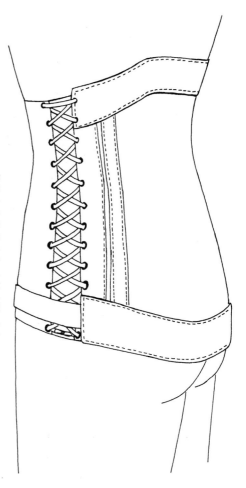

FIGURE 64. LUMBOSACRAL CHAIR-
BACK BRACE

This is a metal and leather or plastic
brace. A pelvic band is located between
the iliac crest and the greater trochanter and is attached by posterior and lateral upright steel struts to a low thoracic
band. Firm abdominal compression is
applied through the laced front "corset" attachment. This brace is heavier
and more rigid but cooler than a corset.
Close fitting of the pelvic and thoracic
bands is crucial for stability and comfort. It is indicated in refractory painful
low back problems. Its chief advantage,
other than durability, may be in restricting lateral flexion. **See page 124.**

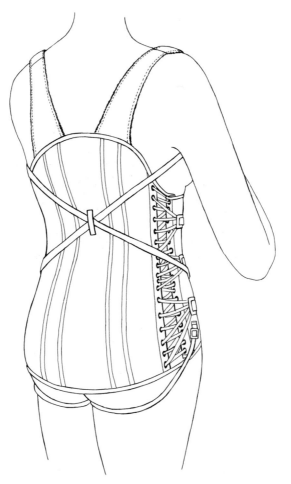

FIGURE 65. THORACO-LUMBAR CORSET

This is a fabric corset with adjustable lacing and elastic components to permit snugness of fit. It is reinforced by stays to increase rigidity. This corset extends from beneath the lower curve of the buttocks to the mid-scapular area and is held in place superiorly by shoulder straps. The use of a mesh fabric improves ventilation; however, in warm climates a long spinal (Taylor) brace may be preferred. These corsets are useful in generalized osteoporosis, in dorsal spinal compression fractures (regardless of etiology), and in painful osteoarthrosis of the dorsal or dorso-lumbar spine. **See page 124.**

ASSISTIVE DEVICES

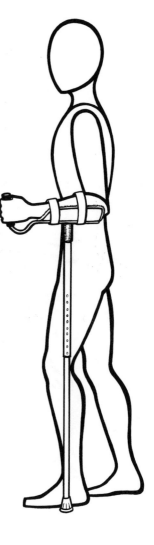

FIGURE 66. Platform crutch

The design of this crutch minimizes stress on wrists and elbows because of the distribution of the body weight over the entire forearm. Stress on finger joints is further minimized by thickened handles and, more importantly, because these handles are primarily used during gait to lift the unweighted crutch. **See Case I. See pages 98 and 129.**

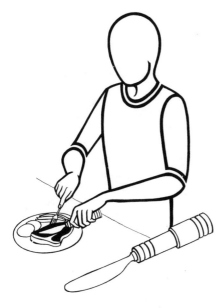

FIGURE 67. Thick-handled knife

Dining and cooking utensils modified to facilitate grasp can be simply fabricated and many are readily available commercially. **See Case I. See page 98.**

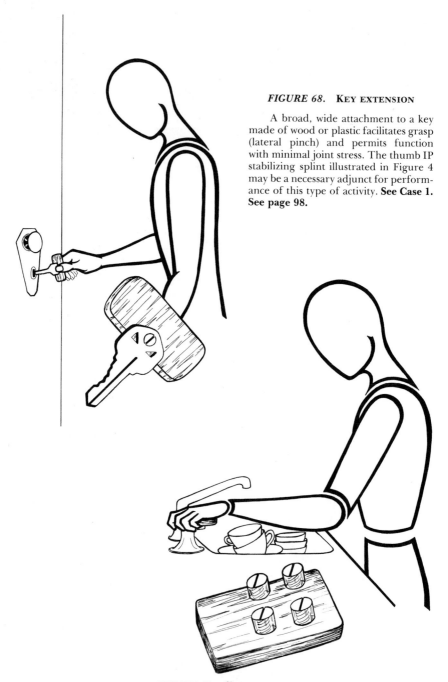

FIGURE 68. Key extension

A broad, wide attachment to a key made of wood or plastic facilitates grasp (lateral pinch) and permits function with minimal joint stress. The thumb IP stabilizing splint illustrated in Figure 4 may be a necessary adjunct for performance of this type of activity. **See Case 1. See page 98.**

FIGURE 69. Faucet lever

A commercially available or easily fabricated device provides increased leverage to facilitate a common household task and to minimize hand and wrist joint stress. The use of bathroom and kitchen fixtures constructed with lever-activated faucets obviates the need for this device. **See Case 1. See page 98.**

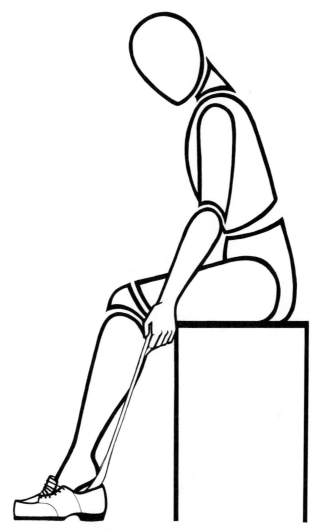

FIGURE 70. **LONG-HANDLED SHOE HORN**

A simple, but too often overlooked, device that can substitute independence and comfort in dressing for agony and the need for assistance. This long-handled shoe horn may be useful for patients with neck, back, or knee joint distress. **See Cases 11, 13 and 15. See page 98.**

Note that elastic shoelaces which do not require tying will stretch sufficiently to permit insertion of the foot but provide enough tension to hold the shoe in place.

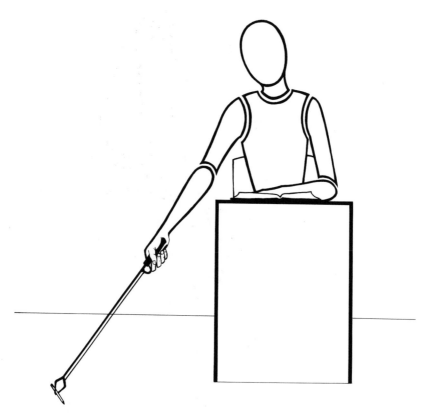

FIGURE 71. REACHER

This is one of several similar devices that permit patients sufficient grasp or reach to compensate for inability to bend down to recover dropped objects or to obtain objects from what would otherwise be inaccessible storage space. **See Cases 1, 5, and 15. See page 98.**

Chapter 4

JOINT PROTECTION

Energy Conservation, Posture, and Joint Positioning

There is usually more than one way to accomplish almost any given task. The conveniences in our modern home and work environments are silent tribute to the effort and expense our society is willing to put forth for convenience and human energy conservation (at the expense of other forms of energy). For the patient with muscular weakness and impaired cardiovascular function, energy conservation is not a matter of convenience alone but is essential to his or her ability to function effectively. It serves little good for a patient to be able to accomplish a given task, e.g., walk up a flight of stairs, only to reach the top utterly exhausted or in pain, and incapable of further effective function. The person who is exhausted, weakened, or pained by a given task is less able to perform the task in question or subsequent activities efficiently and is therefore more vulnerable to accidents or to the imposition of traumatic stresses on arthritic joints.[235]

There are two overriding *principles to be observed in joint protection and energy conservation* for patients with rheumatic diseases: (1) Use large joints with large muscles to protect them in preference to small joints — e.g., carry a handbag with the handle slung over the forearm rather than grasped by the hand. (2) Perform activities so that gravity stresses are minimized — e.g., place heavier objects at table height and slide them toward you rather than lifting them.[113]

Cordery, in a classic discussion, has listed the following precepts for joint protection:

1. *Encourage each joint to be used at a maximum range of motion and strength consistent with the disease process.* This encourages tolerated functional exercise during daily activities.

2. *Avoid positions of deformity, external pressures, and internal stresses.* Pushing off from a bed using the radial side of the hand (external stress)

97

or by forcefully grasping a small handle (internal stress) predisposes to ulnar deviation of the MCP joints.

3. *Use each joint in its most stable anatomical and functional plane.* The use of a platform crutch handle protects the wrist and elbow.

4. *Use the strongest joints available for any given activity.* Carry a purse on a shoulder strap or with handle looped over the forearm to protect the hands and wrists.

5. *Avoid muscle imbalance.* The deforming forces of muscle imbalance resulting from arthritis may require positioning splinting as well as selected exercises as countermeasures during activity. Forced grasping of a small-handled object causes long finger flexor and interosseous muscle predominance, predisposing the hand to ulnar deviating forces.

6. *Any activity that involves holding joints or using muscles in a position for any undue length of time is contraindicated.*

7. The patient should *never attempt an activity that cannot be stopped immediately if it proves to be beyond his power to complete it.*

8. *Respect pain.*[236]

Cordery further suggests the application of the therapeutic approach incorporating these principles:

A. "Reduce the force necessary to accomplish the activity." An example is the use of an oversized handle on an eating utensil or garden tool to avoid the stress to small joints that occurs with tight grasp.

B. "Change the method, sometimes choosing the lesser of evils." Examples are: sliding rather than lifting objects in the kitchen; squeezing water from a sponge by pressing with the palm, rather than using hand grasp; holding a pan by the sides with two hands rather than on the handle with one; turning on a faucet by cupping the palms of both hands around the faucet handle, using the pressure of the heels of the palms to turn it.

C. "Use equipment if necessary." Here the use of supporting splints, braces, reaching devices, long-handled tools, doorknob and faucet levers, refrigerator door and cabinet loops, elevated toilet seats, grab bars, powered can openers, electric or "rocker" knives, canes, crutches, and wheelchairs are useful examples.[236] (See Figs. 66 to 71.)

The intelligent patient, preferably guided by a skilled occupational therapist, can have access to an ever-expanding assortment of items to assist in the various activities of daily living. These items (referenced below) include specially adapted toileting equipment, eating utensils, television and telephonic modifications, equipment to facilitate dressing as well as clothing specially designed for ease of application. Also included are suggestions for modifying household and work environments to enhance accessibility and ease of function. Notable are the placement of ramps over stairs; the use of elevators; and creating work arrangements with a choice of lightweight equipment and tools with modified handle thickness or length to facilitate function; proper desk or table height adjustments and the use of power adaptations where needed.[31, 236-246]

Implicit in the effectiveness of any energy conservation and joint protection program is the emphasis on scheduling and arranging of activities to avoid general fatigue or fatigue to local diseased joint areas. The patient should be taught to perform tasks when seated if possible and with the work space arranged to minimize joint stress. An important contribution of the occupational therapist is to help the patient organize his or her activities and chores so that they are spread out over a period of time and performed in segments interrupted by rest or non-stressful activity in order to minimize stress to joints and general fatigue.

POSTURE, POSITION AND BODY MECHANICS

A general concept of what is "good posture" has been inculcated into all of us, even though the specifics of how to advise patients with regard to the proper standing, sitting, walking, and various work postures are seldom built into our therapeutic armamentarium. The basis for posture recommendations is the desirability of maintaining skeletal alignment in such a way as to minimize articular, muscular, and ligamentous stresses and to maintain maximum mobility for function.[247]

The key to proper body alignment and *correct posture when standing* is preservation of the center of gravity in the center of the body axis.[248] Thus a plumb line from the external auditory meatus (centering the skull) should transect the lateral tip of the acromion, the greater trochanter of the femur, the midpoint of the lateral aspect of the knee, and reach the lateral malleolus or just anterior to it. With "good posture" the dorsal spine kyphosis is modest and the scapulae are positioned to prevent "round shoulders." The pelvis is tilted posteriorly sufficient to minimize the lumbar lordotic curve. A normal adult should be able to stand with his heels 3 to 4 inches from a wall and posteriorly rotate his pelvis (pelvic tilt) so that his occiput, dorsal and lumbar spine, and buttocks are all touching the wall.

The frontal alignment should have the head centered and shoulders level and should show no exaggerated valgus or varus of the knee, or equinus, varus or valgus, of the foot, as evidenced by the ability to approximate both the medial femoral condyles and medial malleoli when standing. Keeping the center of gravity in the midline produces the least stress and therefore requires only minimal muscular effort to maintain the standing posture. Proper posture mitigates against excessive tonic posture-sustaining muscular contractions that can result in muscular strain, pain, muscular fatigue, and articular and periarticular stress.[228, 249, 250]

Optimal *posture for sitting* is determined by the tasks to be performed while seated. The desirable seated position varies and can include that required for close work bent over a desk, sustained tense sitting in conference, relaxed reading, sitting semi-reclined in a rest position, driving, or sitting on a stool for household or shop activities.[112, 229] The overriding consideration in all of these seated activities is alignment of the spine in a manner that will minimize skeletal stress. Thus sitting on a low, soft couch with the legs extended creates excessive posterior tilting of the pelvis and strain from hamstring muscle tension. Alternatively, when one sits in a straight-backed chair that does not allow room posteriorly for buttock protrusion or on an ill-fitted secretarial chair with the lumbar pad position creating a fulcrum that is too high or too low so that it accentuates lumbar lordosis, the result again is low back strain.[112, 228, 229, 250, 251] (See Fig. 51.)

Other considerations in sitting posture are desk height, neck position, and shoulder and elbow angles, as well as the amount of illumination (which will influence the amount of muscle stress in the neck and back needed to assist in visual accommodation).[249-251] Hip and knee mobility become factors in facilitating transfer from sitting to standing and may need accommodation for patients with fixed contractures during sitting or reclining. (Special chairs have been designed for patients with ankylosing spondylitis.)[249-251] For patients who are chair-bound or subject to prolonged sitting, provision should be made for the feet to be firmly planted on a stool or on the floor at a 90-degree angle in order to prevent Achilles tendon shortening.[249-251]

Posture considerations apply not only to sitting and standing but to lying as well. A soft yielding mattress for the patient in the recumbent posture will produce prolonged static stresses on muscular and ligamentous structures, and this is further aggravated when the support (box spring or bed boards) underlying the mattress itself sags. The patient who sits semi-propped in bed, with the dorsal spine rounded, the neck bent forward, the hips flexed, the knees flexed, and the feet plantar-flexed, is putting his body at a maximum disadvantage unless these abnormal postures are compensated by appropriate positioning and exercise. The pillow under the arthritic knee is a notorious culprit in the genesis of hip and knee flexion contractures.[154]

A flexion contracture of the knee means that the angle of the femur and tibia is such that the quadriceps muscle must continuously contract in order to maintain the standing position. This posture increases intra-articular knee stress and taxes a quadriceps muscle already weakened by the condition that led to the contracture, and thereby reduces ambulation tolerance, frequently necessitating the employment of a cane or crutches for safe, sustained ambulation.

A hip flexion contracture must be compensated for either by lumbar lordo-sis or by knee flexion. Lumbar lordosis is almost always compromised by ankylosing spondylitis or in the geriatric population by advanced discogenic disease. In order to remain erect with a hip flexion con-tracture and a stiff spine, flexion must occur at the knee. This creates additional stresses on the knee and a mechanically inefficient gait be-cause of the functional shortening in the contractured leg.[142, 154]

Positioning should be used therapeutically to prevent contractures by utilizing well-designed furniture, minimal pillows, firm mattresses, and bedboards and by encouraging prone positioning to compensate for the tendency for hip flexion contractures to develop in patients who spend a great deal of time in bed, or in a seated position when out of bed.[112, 113, 154, 229]

Of equal importance to static posture considerations is the *teach-ing of proper body mechanics.* Patients may need to learn methods to facilitate arising and reclining from and to a horizontal position in bed, or arising from or lowering to a chair, as well as how to stand (one foot on a low stool reduces lumbosacral stress) so as to minimize musculoskeletal strain. (See Figs. 40 to 42.)[113, 249, 250, 252] Dynamic as-pects of postural considerations in the lower extremity and trunk are crucial to patients with low back pain and discogenic disease and care-ful instruction in proper body mechanics to minimize stress on sitting and standing can be an important determining factor in the success of therapy and even to the patient's ultimate return to vocational activi-ty.[112, 229, 235, 250, 251]

It is well recognized that bending over to pick up a heavy object can maximally load the lumbar disks. What is often overlooked is that the process of bending over, even to pick up a paper napkin, creates a significant disk stress and that this may be greatly compounded by the torque associated with a rotary movement. The result of an apparent-ly innocuous movement can result in severe stress to the vulnerable fibers of the annulus fibrosus in the lumbar disks.[228, 249, 250, 253-257]

Where weakness and contractures impose postural problems that preclude independent standing and ambulation, bracing and the use of ambulation assistive devices, as discussed below, are necessary to compensate for the functional deficiency.

Posture per se is less crucial than positioning where the upper extremities are concerned. Improper seating can lead to shortening of the pectoral muscles as a consequence of chair arm rests that are placed either too high or too close. This can also predispose to malpo-sition of the elbows, wrists, and ultimately fingers. The interdepen-dent linking mechanism in the joints of the upper extremities is more apparent than in those of the lower extremities. *In the rheumatoid ar-thritis patient with multiple joint involvement, a loss of mobility in any one joint leads to increased stress on those joints required to compensate for the lost motion.* Unfortunately these joints are all too often compromised as well by the arthritic process. A painful arthritic knee may necessitate the use of crutches for ambulation, but the crutches may require modification or even prove impractical because of finger, wrist, elbow, and shoulder involvement.

During acute, severe, generalized arthritic exacerbations and even more particularly in the face of a septic arthritic process, effective prophylactic joint range of motion exercise may be near impossible because of pain and swelling. The goals of therapy may then be restricted to minimizing deformity by optimal positioning and gentle mobilizing exercises, if tolerated, to preserve as much range of motion as possible. (See Table 3-1.)

SELECTED READINGS BY TOPICS

(See also complete Bibliography on page 213.)

Joint Protection, Energy Conservation

236. Cordery, J.: The conservation of physical resources as applied to the activities of patients with arthritis and the connective tissue diseases. Study Course III, Third International Congress, World Federation of Occupational Therapists. Dubuque, Iowa: William C. Brown Co., 1962. P. 22.
237. Accent on Living, Inc. Gillum Road and High Drive, P.O. Box 700, Bloomington, Illinois 61701. n.d.
238. May, E. E., Waggoner, N. R., Hotte, E. B.: *Independent Living for the Handicapped and the Elderly.* Boston: Houghton Mifflin Company, 1974, Pp. 120, 251.
239. Lowman, E. W., Klinger, J. L.: *Aids to Independent Living; Self-Help for the Handicapped.* New York: McGraw-Hill, Inc., 1969.
245. Talbot, B.: "Chapter 27. Automobile modifications for disabled," *in* S. Licht, H. Kamenetz, eds., *Orthotics Etcetera.* New Haven: E. Licht, 1966. P. 676.

Posture

247. Hines, T. F.: "Chapter 20. Posture," *in* S. Licht, ed., *Therapeutic Exercise.* 2nd Ed. Baltimore: Waverly Press, 1965. P. 486.
249. Kendall, H. O., Kendall, F. P., Boynton, D. A.: *Posture and Pain.* Baltimore: Williams and Wilkins, 1952.
250. Eklundh, M.: *Spare Your Back.* London: Gerald Duckworth Co., Ltd., 1966.
251. Keegan, J. J.: Alterations of lumbar curve related to posture and seating. J. Bone Joint Surg., *35A:* 589, July 1953.
255. Nachemson, A., Elfström, G.: *Intravital Dynamic Pressure Measurements in Lumbar Discs; a Study of Common Movements, Maneuvers and Exercises.* Stockholm: Almqvist & Wiksell, 1970.

Chapter 5

SPLINTS, BRACES, SHOES AND CORSETS

SPLINTING AND BRACING: GENERAL CONSIDERATIONS

In appearance, splints and braces can be deceptively simple. Their proper selection and design, however, may require the utmost in sophistication, not only in regard to assessing the clinical indications for their application but also with respect to the bioengineering technology and the evaluation of their functional efficacy. A splint or brace must be precisely chosen to meet a specific clinical indication. This may be to position and stabilize an extremity, to minimize pain or to increase function, or it may involve the application of corrective forces to prevent or correct a deformity.

Choice of materials is determined by the task the splint or brace must perform and consideration must be given to durability, weight, tissue irritation and allergy, resistance to deformation, hygiene, cosmesis, ease of fabrication and modification, and cost.[258]

A splint or brace must be designed so that it may be applied, adjusted or removed by the wearer without assistance whenever possible. It should cause no constriction, blanching, edema, numbness, or abrasion. A shorthand guideline to gauge the effectiveness of a splint or brace stipulates that when the patient returns for a follow-up visit the splint or brace shows significant evidence of wear. This criterion does not satisfy a number of important orthotic considerations.[259] What is the value of the specific splint or brace as opposed to alternative designs? Is it a solution to more than short-term goals? Is the functional objective of the splint achieved, and if so at what cost in terms of other functional or psychosocial maladaptations?[259]

The issue of *proper alignment of splints and braces is crucial* to effective splinting or bracing in many instances.[260] Examples of problems with malalignment are the inability to flex the MCP joints when a wrist-stabilizing splint is extended beyond the distal palmar crease

103

(this may be prescribed intentionally to provide a stretch stimulus to tight intrinsics), the potential of a lumbar spinal brace for accentuating painful lumbar lordosis by improper adaptation to the pelvis, or the compression of neurovascular structures of the thigh and calf by malalignment of the knee hinge in long leg braces.[261-264]

A basic biomechanical consideration in splinting and bracing is the proper application of the *three-point pressure principle,* in which two points of pressure at the extremes of the brace are resisted by one point of counterpressure either to achieve stability, where that is the object, or to provide a correcting counterforce when treating a deformity.[263] Inappropriate alignment of pressure-counterpressure couples can lead to shear stresses that are transferred to the brace, causing increasing wear, and, more importantly, stress on the underlying tissues and resultant deformity — a problem particularly crucial to the growing child.[263, 264] The stresses imposed on the brace are not limited to the brace mechanism or soft tissue and bone. In lower extremity bracing, stresses are imposed on the foot and the shoe that contains it. A properly fitting, sturdy orthopedic shoe is crucial to the successful application of any brace fitted on the shoe.

With the exceptions of postoperative positioning and contracture correction, there is no solid evidence that splints or braces lead to reversal of arthritis-caused malalignments. Prevention of progression of deformities is a reasonable objective, but the choice of method and approach requires experience and judgment. Therefore, the *temptation by therapists or orthotists inexperienced in the management of arthritic problems to attempt corrective splinting or bracing should be strongly resisted* **unless the splint or brace serves to relieve pain or improve function.**

As in the case of adaptive equipment, no matter how cleverly a device or splint may seem to solve a problem, *in the final analysis it is the patient's toleration for gadgets and equipment that determines whether or not they will be used.* If a patient complains that a device or splint or brace is uncomfortable or interferes with function, the device should probably be modified or abandoned — and, in fact, it probably will be by the patient. (See Table 5–1, *Useful Splints and Braces.*)

SPLINTING TO REDUCE INFLAMMATION

The utilization of splints to *maintain inflamed or weakened joints in positions of function* is well established, and the beneficial effect of splinting or casting to immobilize joints in order to relieve inflammation has also been well documented.[104, 108, 265-268] The consensus is that a rheumatoid arthritic joint *will usually demonstrate a lessening of pain and inflammation after immobilization for two to four weeks and is unlikely to develop a fixed contracture.*[104, 108, 267]

TABLE 5-1. Useful Splints and Braces*

Region	Indication	Purpose	Type	Reference
Hand	Acute inflammation	Stability for pain relief Preservation of position for function	Volar resting splint** to include forearm and fingers in position of function	285
Thumb	CMC & MCP joint arthritis	Stabilize for pain relief, permit function	Thumb post with wrist strap	285
	De Quervain's tenosynovitis	Relieve pain	Thumb post with wrist strap	285
	IP joint pain or instability	Improve function, relieve pain	Thumb IP "sleeve" or "double ring"	287
Wrists	Active inflammation	Improve function, relieve pain	Static "working" wrist splint***	285
	Instability	Improve function, relieve pain	Static "working" wrist splint	
	Carpal tunnel syndrome	Prevent hyperflexion and nerve compression	Static "working" wrist splint	
Knee	Pain, instability	Pain relief Maintain position during weight bearing	Long leg, hinged knee with lock	305
Ankle, hind foot	Pain on weight bearing	Support foot and relieve weight bearing stress	Cushion heel, rocker sole, below knee weight bearing brace	313
Forefoot	Pain on weight bearing	Support foot and relieve weight bearing stress	Metatarsal pad/bar	316

*Postoperative splints not included.
**Resting splints maximally support affected joints, usually at sacrifice of function.
***Static working splints stabilize affected joints but permit maximum function (See Figure 52). Dynamic splints provide wire or elastic tension for traction or to assist weak muscles. Various dynamic splints (wire and/or rubber band–assisted traction devices) are employed to maintain postoperative corrections. The Bunnell "knuckle bender" splints are occasionally helpful in treating an isolated finger contracture where inflammation is minimal. Splints for thumb IP stabilization to correct swan neck, boutonniere, or ulnar deviation deformities are available, but their efficacy is unproved.

CASTING TO OVERCOME CONTRACTURES

The role of casting as a means of overcoming contractures is largely confined to flexion contractures of the knee, although it can be used in the elbow and wrist as well.[109, 142, 143, 149, 269, 270] Painful contractured joints supported in a position of extension in a cast become less painful and are no longer restricted by protective flexor muscle contraction. The relaxation of the flexor muscles allows for gradual stretching to occur within the cast. Immobilization reduces inflammation and swelling and thereby potentiates the effectiveness of the cast as a stretching modality.

SERIAL KNEE CASTING

The cast can consist of a cylinder extending from the upper thigh to just above the malleoli, changed every five to seven days, or a molded posterior shell extending from the upper thigh to include the foot (placed in a neutral position) and reaching beyond the tips of the toes or, alternatively, a full cast bisected at the angle of the joint and wedged 1 to 2 degrees per day by means of turnbuckle screw-adjusting hinges or bending irons inserted in the plaster.[109, 149, 269] The use of serial wedge casts is generally impractical with knee flexion contractures of greater than 45 degrees, and traction is then preferred. With wedging casts there is risk of abutment and compression of the posteriorly subluxing tibia onto the femur, but this problem can be minimized with proper positioning or by the use of traction.[142, 143]

To facilitate maximal leg extension before application of the cast, the patient can be placed prone.[143] The plaster is then applied directly to the skin and carefully molded without any protective interface, and with cuffs placed above and below the knee, leaving the remainder of the leg and foot open.[143] In this method the distal cuff is split after approximately five days and, if the heel can be lifted from the shell, sufficient extension has been obtained to require application of another cast.[143] Using any of these methods with approximately four to five castings or 1 or 2 degrees of wedging daily, one can ultimately achieve a knee extension of 10 degrees or less in the majority of cases.[143, 149]

The risk of loss of flexion in prolonged casting, as previously mentioned, has been shown to be minimal if the cast is removed approximately every four to five days and the patient put through a range of motion or, preferably, if the cast is bivalved and the leg removed for range of motion as well as strengthening exercises daily. Whenever possible, the patient who has been successfully treated for flexion contracture of the knee should ambulate with the use of crutches, cane, or a long leg brace until such time as quadriceps function is sufficient to maintain the leg in extension during ambulation.

POSITIONS OF FUNCTION

SHOULDER

In all joints the position of least tension for the capsule is somewhere in mid-range of motion.[271, 272] This position of partial flexion (or elevation in the shoulder) is also the antalgic or least painful position for the joint.[133, 218, 271-279] With the use of heat for pain relief, one can often position the shoulder in a bed rest position in abduction and external rotation, alternating with full shoulder flexion (the forearm alongside the ear with the elbow either flexed or extended). Because of the stretch it imposes on the capsule this position may not be tolerated. However, with the support of pillows to resist gravitational stresses and with the use of hot or cold packs for pain relief, one can often achieve a resting position that minimizes the most deleterious aspects of severe shoulder contractures or the so-called "frozen" shoulder.

The problem of contractures in the shoulder is not only a concern for patients with inflammatory or septic arthritis but occurs as a consequence of periarticular disorders, including tendinitis, bursitis, the so-called shoulder-hand syndrome, trauma, and as a complication of disuse in patients with polymyositis and other neuromuscular paralytic disorders. The strategy of positioning to minimize contracture or as a means of a gentle stretching therapy, therefore, has wide application.

If ankylosis of the glenohumeral joint is unavoidable, *the optimal functional position* for an immobile shoulder is one that will permit the hand to get to the top of the head for grooming (and thus for feeding as well) and also be available for tasks such as buttoning shirts and tucking in shirttails or blouses. Forty-five degrees of abduction, 15 degrees of flexion and 15 degrees of internal rotation of the humerus on the scapula at the glenohumeral joint are recommended for females to accomplish these objectives. These figures are increased by 10 degrees in abduction and flexion in males in order to facilitate more vigorous activities.[280]

ELBOW

The untreated arthritic elbow will usually assume a position of partial flexion in mid-range between pronation and supination. The loss of elbow extension does not pose a serious problem except as it is compounded by restriction of motion in other joints in the upper extremity linkage. Far more serious is the loss of elbow flexion because if the elbow cannot flex beyond 90 degrees one has great difficulty in feeding, grooming, or even in scratching one's face. To preserve extension in early active arthritis, a posterior molded resting splint (Plastazote is easily molded for this purpose) accompanied by range of motion exercises to minimize restriction of flexion is useful. In the occasional patient, gentle traction to overcome flexion or extension contractures of the elbow by means of a dynamic splint, consisting of a wrist and an upper arm cuff bridged by rubber bands or a spring wire, worn intermittently for 20 to 30 minutes at a time, merits a few weeks of trial.

If a permanent contracture of the elbow is a likely outcome, consideration must be given to the function in the opposite upper extremity. Fortunately, it is unusual for a total loss of elbow flexion to occur, but when this is inevitable, fixation of an elbow at 70 degrees of flexion (in unilateral elbow involvement) will usually prove to be the optimal position of function, barring modifications required by the patient's activities of daily living and the functional capabilities of the other joints in both upper and lower extremities.[281] Where both elbows will become fixed, an angle of 70 degrees in one and 150 degrees in the other is recommended.[281, 270] (See Table 3–1.)

WRIST

The wrist cannot be thought of in isolation, particularly when it is involved as part of a generalized arthritic process. It is recognized that for optimal grasp strength the lengthening effect on the finger flexors caused by moderate dorsal flexion at the wrist is essential. This has led to widespread acknowledgment that dorsiflexion is the optimal position for wrist function.[151, 270] In the rheumatoid, where both wrists and other joints are involved, there may be great disadvantages to this position because of the inconvenience it causes during writing and toileting (wiping), not to mention the lack of likelihood that a powerful hand grasp can be employed. Other considerations in the rheumatoid hand are the strong metacarpophalangeal subluxating and ulnar deviating torque that is increased by forces occurring during hand grasp and by radial carpal deviation.[132] Hence, in a rheumatoid, if a wrist is to be fused or immobilized in a position of function, the neutral position is generally chosen. If both wrists must be fused or splinted in a position of optimal function, the nondominant one may be more functional in 5 to 10 degrees of palmar flexion and ulnar deviation to facilitate personal hygiene.[150] (See Table 3–1.) Specific indications for wrist and hand splinting including selection of materials, patterns for fabrication and sources of materials have been compiled in a useful manual.[258]

HAND

Positioning the hand for maximum function where motion cannot be maintained requires that the MCP joints of the fingers be placed in 30 to 40 degrees of flexion, the PIP joints in 35 degrees of flexion, the thumb carpometacarpal joint rotated and abducted 40 to 60 degrees, the thumb MCP joint placed in 20 degrees of flexion and 15 degrees of internal rotation and adduction, and the thumb IP joint made straight, provided pre-existing deformities and functional problems do not otherwise dictate.[150, 282, 283] (See Table 3–1.)

KNEE AND HIP

Because of the importance of a straight leg in standing and ambulation (let alone the difficulties that occur with severe hip and knee flexion contractures in attempting to roll over in bed or to lie prone) the optimal position for a stiff knee to facilitate a free swinging gait and prevent tripping on the foot is from 10 to 20 degrees of flexion.[284] (See Table 3–1.) During acute or chronic inflammatory involvement of the knee where there is an incipient or overt flexion contracture, resting splints to maintain the knee in full extension, or serial casts or wedged casts to correct existing contractures are employed, as discussed previously.[109, 143, 149, 269]

Since the advent of the total hip arthroplasty, fusion of the hip has become less common. Where ankylosis is inevitable the hip is generally most functional for ambulation, and reasonably functional for sitting and self-care, if it is in 20 to 30 degrees of flexion, 5 degrees of abduction, and slight internal rotation.[282] (See Table 3–1.)

ANKLE

With a patient supine, the weight and tension of sheets and bed coverings on the unprotected foot predispose it to plantar flexion contracture, and prolonged prone positioning of the patient will have the same effect unless the foot is extended over the end of the mattress. The optimum position of the ankle at rest is in midposition or in 10 degrees of plantar flexion for women who prefer higher heels.[270] (See Table 3–1.) For the patient in bed with acute arthritis, this position can be achieved by use of a foot board, or better, by the use of a short leg splint with foot support, or the extension of a posterior molded knee splint or brace to enclose the foot with the ankle positioned at a 90 degree angle to the leg. Heel lifts and specially designed shoes can compensate for an abnormal ankle position, and surgery can be employed to correct severe plantar flexion ankle deformities. For the patient who does not want an operation and finds it difficult to put on shoes at night in order to be able to walk to the lavatory, it is desirable to avoid the problem entirely with proper positioning and exercise.

SPECIFIC "ESTABLISHED" INDICATIONS FOR SPLINTING OR BRACING FOR PATIENTS WITH ARTHRITIS OF THE WRIST AND HAND

The crucial importance of hand function and the impact of the cosmetic effects of hand deformity on the arthritis sufferer have stimulated many attempts to correct hand deformity, relieve pain, or improve function by splinting or bracing. Splints are fabricated in a variety of materials including plastic, plaster of paris, cloth, leather, and metal.[285, 286] Metal has the advantage of being lightweight and durable and in certain applications can be designed so as to eliminate buckles and clips that can be difficult to apply and tend to stretch, break, or undergo deterioration.[287-290]

The popular thermolabile plastic materials have various characteristics and advantages and disadvantages. The high-temperature materials (Nyloplex, Royalite, and Kydex) require power tools for cutting and must be formed over a positive mold of the region to be splinted. They are rigid and can be used in warm water without deforming but are more difficult to fit precisely. The low-temperature materials (Orthoplast, San-Splint Plastazote, Prenyl) can be cut with scissors and heated and molded directly on the patient. They are less rigid, deform when exposed to heat (cannot be worn when washing dishes in a sink), and tend to become soiled easily.[258] The choice of material depends on the indication, preferences and skill of the fabricator, and cost, but the widespread use of low-temperature materials suggests that their practical advantages outweigh their disadvantages. The ease of fabrication of hand orthoses with thermolabile plastic materials has made readily available simple, lightweight, cosmetically acceptable splints, but by the same token has made fabrication so simple that the temptation to provide splints often exceeds the indications.[258, 285, 286]

As previously discussed under *splinting,* the use of a so-called *resting hand splint* to immobilize the entire hand and wrist, as well as the volar surface of the bulk of the forearm, *is indicated only in rare instances* to stabilize a very severely inflamed hand, as might be found in a case of sepsis, crystal-induced arthritis, or an occasional severe, acute, uncontrolled rheumatoid or variant inflammation.[258, 285] When used bilaterally, resting hand splints preclude hand function and make impossible even the simple, yet important, task of pulling on covers for warmth.

On the other hand, a *static ("working") wrist splint* designed to stabilize a wrist that is painful, inflamed, and volarly subluxed, or to minimize compression of the median nerve in a carpal tunnel syndrome, while not protective of finger joints, permits hand function and has had wide acceptance.[141, 150, 258, 285] Where the wrist-stabilizing or working splint is applied to prevent inflammation and swelling, it should be worn during daily activities. The unavoidable encroachment of these splints on the proximal portion of the palm may interfere with certain kinds of grasping activities, such as holding a broomstick. The patient will determine for himself the extent, if any, that the splint may interfere with function in a specific task, but most activities of daily living and housekeeping chores can be accomplished with the working wrist splint in place.[141, 258, 285] (See Fig. 52.)

Custom-fitted plastic splints are generally preferable, but commercially available metal-reinforced fabric splints are often effective and economical. Commercial plastic or metal splints rarely fit properly, often require considerable modification, and are generally excessively bulky. For severe carpal tunnel syndromes, particularly in association with inflammation of the wrist, the working splint should be worn during the day and night. However, many patients with carpal tunnel syndrome are distressed by malposition of the wrist only during sleep, and thus wearing the splint only at night will suffice (Fig. 52).

The characteristic and distressing *ulnar deviation deformity* of the rheumatoid hand challenges the therapeutic creativity of all who must attempt to cope with it. The dynamics of the deforming forces in the rheumatoid hand have been recently reviewed and the significance of the stresses occurring during grasp on the inflamed metacarpophalangeal joints as the major causal factor in ulnar deviation have been delineated.[132, 291, 292]

The keys to prevention or correction of ulnar deviation would appear to be restricting flexion and ulnar deviation in the MCP joints, preventing ulnar deviation of the fifth MCP joint, and correction of radial deviation of the carpi.[132, 292] Splints have been devised that meet these criteria, but their value in preventing or correcting ulnar deviation has not been established.[258, 289, 293-295] The use of splints to prevent or correct ulnar deviating deformities per se is at this time experimental and splints should be prescribed for this purpose only with the constraints of a carefully controlled study. *Positioning splints that correct ulnar deviation are justifiably applied to patients where they improve cosmesis* to the patient's satisfaction or *enhance hand comfort and function.*[258, 287] The author's personal preference is a simple positioning splint designed to resist ulnar deviation–MCP flexion forces while restricting ulnar deviating movement of the MCP joints and still permit useful hand function. (See Fig. 53.)[294]

Dynamic splints using rubber band tension, while useful in correcting alignment during postoperative scar formation, have been shown to be of no value in correcting ulnar deviation in the nonsurgical management of rheumatoid arthritis.[150, 281, 296-298]

Similar problems and temptations occur in efforts to correct the *swan neck* and *boutonnière* finger deformities as well as instability of thumb joints in the rheumatoid hand.[132] Bennett has described useful splints made of metal for stabilization of the thumb either at the IP joint or MCP joint.[289] (See Fig. 54.) For *swan neck deformities* he advocates splints designed to restrict the PIP hyperextension deformity while permitting flexion of the PIP joints.[289] These splints can be fabricated in thermolabile plastic materials as well.[289] When such splints are worn on adjacent fingers they tend to catch on one another, but in selected cases they can enhance stability of the proximal interphalangeal joint while permitting useful flexion.

Dynamic splints using gentle rubber band tension on spring wire devices (Bunnell knuckle benders) for a few weeks are particularly useful in postoperative management and are occasionally effective in overcoming an isolated flexion or extension contracture in a finger joint.[150, 281, 298] (See Figs. 7 and 8.) Their efficacy in overcoming contracture in patients with progressive systemic sclerosis is not established. Regardless of the indications, if dynamic splints are used, precise measurements of the joints to be stretched should be made. The duration of application of tension should be restricted or timed so as not to aggravate the joint disease. Twenty to 30 minute sessions every two to four hours when awake[281] are usually tolerated, but 60 minute sessions with careful supervision of adjustments of tension may be more efficient. If measurable changes are not demonstrable within two weeks, or if after initial improvement no progress is noted by measurement on two successive weekly evaluations, or if joint symptoms are consistently exacerbated by the use of the splint, splinting should be discontinued.

In the case of *boutonnière* deformities or in flexion contractures of the PIP joints, the role of splinting is less sure. The functional consequences of restricting PIP flexion during activity (when the deforming forces are operative) usually preclude their acceptance by the patient. Their effectiveness if worn only intermittently or at rest is not established. In the management of boutonnière deformities the value of a functional splint designed to restrict PIP flexion partially rather than completely has not been reported.

In osteoarthritis of the *thumb*, involvement of the first carpometacarpal joint, or less commonly of the metacarpophalangeal joint, may cause considerable pain and weakness on pinch or grasp. This can be alleviated in many instances by application of a simple plastic or metal positioning and stabilizing splint that slips over the proximal phalanx of the thumb (leaving the thumb pad exposed for pinch) and extends proximally along the shaft of the first metacarpal and CMC joint, where it is affixed by a wrist strap.[52, 258, 285, 289, 299, 300] (See Fig. 55.)

A similar splint involving a short "thumb post" is a useful adjunct in the management of stenosing tenosynovitis of the long thumb abductor and short thumb extensor (DeQuervain's disease).[258, 285, 300] (See Fig. 55.) It should be noted that a variety of prefabricated hand splints have been designed that have both the advantages and disadvantages of standardization in that they are widely available but in most instances have been designed to correct or compensate for neuromuscular damage rather than management of arthritic disorders.[301]

In an *acute tenosynovitis* of the finger flexors, a resting hand splint with hand and fingers positioned to preserve function may be indicated.[258] In *chronic tenosynovitis* with local "triggering" occurring on full flexion of a PIP joint, a one-inch-wide sewn sleeve of elastic worn over the PIP joint will allow for all but the last 20 or 30 degrees of PIP flexion and may relieve troublesome tendon entrapment and triggering. (See Fig. 57.)

There have been two published reports of uncontrolled studies on the use of *elastic cloth gloves* for the symptomatic treatment of osteoarthritis and rheumatoid arthritis involving the hands.[302, 303] Although subjective improvement was claimed in these reports, no subjective or objective benefit other than slight reduction in ring size in some patients with rheumatoid arthritis was observed in a recent controlled study.[304]

THE ELBOW AND SHOULDER

The use of a resting splint for the acutely inflamed *elbow* can be of value in relieving pain. This is preferably implemented with a posterior shell or gutter splint (Plastazote rather than plaster of paris) with the elbow positioned in approximately 20 degrees of flexion and supination and with provision for the splint to be removed daily for range of motion exercise to preserve flexion.[270] For the occasional patient left with a contracture that limits elbow flexion after elbow inflammation has largely subsided, the use of a dynamic splint, consisting of a proximal arm and wrist cuff with rubberband tension, gently applied for a period of 20 to 30 minutes every two to four hours during the day may be helpful as an adjunct to active-assisted range of motion exercises in restoring elbow flexion.

An exquisitely *painful acute arthritis or bursitis of the shoulder* may be relieved in part by the *use of a supporting arm sling.*

BRACING IN THE LOWER EXTREMITIES

Lower extremity braces have been traditionally made of metal, are bulky, heavy, and where dresses are worn, cosmetically unappealing. These problems have been more than offset by the improvement in stability and function that lower extremity bracing permits when weakness secondary to neuromuscular problems is the primary concern. Lower extremity bracing to relieve painful arthritic conditions has been much less successful, not only in patients with multiple joint involvement who have difficulty using canes or crutches but in patients with isolated hip or knee joint involvement as well.

Leg braces are often difficult for the arthritic patient to put on without assistance. Where the knee requires locking of the brace in extension for stability, consideration must be given to the problems of dexterity necessary for activating the locking mechanism. A rod extension with a loop-ring attachment at the proximal thigh may facilitate locking and unlocking a long leg brace for the patient who cannot bend, reach, or perform pinch function.[305] Unless a brace is properly fitted, the weight-bearing load on the joint that is being braced may not be relieved. Indeed, poor brace alignment across the affected joint may impose additional stress at joints proximal or distal to it.[260, 264, 306-308]

For the patient whose ambulation is markedly limited by a painful arthritic knee, an assessment of the potential efficacy of long leg bracing can be made by the application of a temporary cylinder cast or an adjustable temporary long leg brace.[152] Conventional long leg braces are designed with a hinge at the knee and the ankle, and are stabilized proximally with a thigh cuff (customarily made of leather) with further stability supplied by a patellar pad. Two recent advances in knee orthoses have provided the orthotist with a lightweight plastic, ischial weight-bearing brace with a standard hinged knee that assists ambulation where muscular weakness is the major problem, and a brace designed with only a single upright strut to reduce weight while still providing stability and optimal alignment for the arthritic knee.[264, 309-311] The utilization of plastic orthoses in the spinal cord injured, dystrophic, and hemiparetic patients has been expanding.[307, 308] The application of plastic materials and the principles of their fitting, modified appropriately for arthritic joint problems, should be aggressively explored.

The use of *elastic fabric knee splints,* or "cages," with or without hinges, has not been critically evaluated but they frequently provide sufficient support or at least comfort (by whatever mechanism) to minimize knee joint stress on transfer and during ambulation. The constriction of the leg by the application of elastic splints or bandages may pose problems in patients with circulatory insufficiency.

In summary, splinting the arthritic knee, whether it be for rheumatoid arthritis or degenerative joint disease, may be of value in relieving articular stress but requires careful prescription and design. The location of hinges, straps, and bands and questions related to ease of application and removal by the patient must be considered. In selected patients, particularly where only one extremity is involved, long leg bracing may be of value.

For the occasional patient with chronic *hip pain* not relieved by cane or crutch support, the use of a brace in which the weight is borne on the ischium (pelvis), and therefore above the hip joint, by an *ischial weight-bearing brace* may be of value.[305, 306, 312]

ANKLE AND HIND FOOT

The *ankle and hind foot* are not infrequently the source of persistent and disabling pain on standing or ambulation. These problems can often be obviated by shoe modifications (discussed subsequently), but on occasion a short leg brace is required for functional ambulation. A below-knee weight-bearing brace, which transmits the weight of the body from the heel of the shoe through two upright struts to the upper calf and then distributes the body weight by a plastic or leather cuff over the calf surface, particularly over the upper anterior tibial area below the knee joint, is a useful solution to pain in the ankle and hind foot.[313] (See Fig. 58.)

When the ankle is involved, immobilization of the ankle by elimination of the ankle hinge may be required and ankle motion is then compensated for by means of a "SACH" or cushioned heel and rocker sole.[313] (See Fig. 59.) Experiments with plastic ankle orthoses have been largely confined to compensating for weakness or spasticity associated with paralysis and their effectiveness in stabilizing the arthritic joint has not had adequate trial.[314]

Painful *subtalar joints* and particularly *heel pain* on the anterior calcaneus at the plantar fascial insertion are very disabling problems for the arthritic patient. When all else fails, the below-knee weight-bearing brace, as described above, may offer a somewhat cumbersome but welcome solution, but this is rarely necessary; and there are a number of options that can be tried sequentially before considering a brace.[313] A crepe or ripple sole may provide adequate cushioning and relieve calcaneal distress. If the sole is too soft it creates instability and sheer stresses on walking that can aggravate the local problem or provoke stress on more proximal joints. The use of a padded heel insert, which may be designed in a horseshoe fashion supporting the entire heel except where the open portion of the horseshoe gives clearance for the painful anterior central calcaneus, or as a cover for a hole excavated in the interior of the heel of the shoe into which additional foam rubber is placed, can serve to cushion the sensitive area on the calcaneus.[222] The weight borne on the heel is distributed on the perimeter of the soft tissues overlying the calcaneus and not at the point of irritation on the anterior inner surface. The use of a commercially available plastic heel cup is a simple and often effective means of relieving anterior calcaneal plantar fascia insertion pain, the apparent mechanism being compression of the soft tissue under the heel and redistribution of weight-bearing surfaces.

Arch supports, with or without other heel modifications as described above, are sometimes of value, again apparently by virtue of their ability to distribute some of the weight-bearing load onto the arch support. A more sophisticated and rational approach to anterior calcaneal or heel *"spur"* pain, utilizing the UC-BL plastic molded hind foot shoe insert, was recently described.[141, 315] It should be emphasized that in many patients the use of an occasional local steroid, injection with or without a simple shoe modification or change, may be sufficient to relieve a troublesome plantar fasciitis.

MID-FOOT PROBLEMS

Occasionally the mid-tarsal region is selectively involved in a chronic arthritic process. Key to the management of almost all foot problems is the use of proper supporting footwear. This is particularly true in the mid-tarsal region where a multiply laced shoe (a tennis shoe is often very successful) may provide sufficient well distributed support and stability to relieve painful articular motion in the mid-tarsal joints. A trial of adhesive strapping under the arch and over the dorsum of the foot can help assess the possibilities for benefit from a broad elastic strap or commercially available elastic glove-like foot bandage as a means of providing mid-foot support. The elastic strap can have a laced closure for easy adjustment of tension, but usually a Velcro closure will suffice and requires less space within the shoe to accommodate it.

The ideal shoe to provide foot support for patients whose more proximal weight-bearing joints are involved should have: a rigid steel shank extending longitudinally from the heel to the MTP joint line to support the mid-tarsal "arch" area; a firm well-fitting heel counter to hold the calcaneus in optimal alignment and to prevent the foot from sliding in the shoe; ample width, length, and depth in the toe box to accommodate deformities and to mitigate any abnormal pressure on the foot.[152, 316] The shoe should have a tie lacing with multiple lace holes to allow for wide distribution of the supporting trusses over the dorsum of the foot. The ideal shoe should also have a heel height of approximately one inch, as a higher heel would stress the forefoot, and a lower one the ankle and heel. For the patient with severe involvement of the hands or restriction in reach, elastic shoe laces or Velcro tongue closures may be required to secure the shoe.[316]

There are several commercial shoes, available as prescription footwear, that meet these ideal criteria and have the advantage of sufficient roominess to permit the insertion of custom-molded sole and heel modifications when required. Shoe weight is often a consideration, and the use of sandals or lightweight plastic shoes or tennis shoes may be required where footwear weight is a crucial issue.[317] Oversized tennis shoes provide room and ease of modification with appropriate custom insoles to accommodate the arthritic foot.

FOREFOOT PROBLEMS

The most common disability in the rheumatoid foot is a consequence of metatarsal-phalangeal arthritis. Common nonrheumatoid problems, in addition to the almost ubiquitous osteoarthritis of the first MTP joint, are: metatarsalgia secondary to an abnormally long second metatarsal (Morton's toe), and intermetatarsal neuralgia secondary to compression of the conjoint branches of the medial and lateral plantar nerves proximal to the third and fourth metatarsal heads (Morton's neuroma).

Essential to the treatment of all these problems is *provision of adequate shoe space for the forefoot.* The width of the foot as well as the length of the toes, plus any additional space-occupying problems as a consequence of secondarily cocked up toes, hammer toes, or overlapping toes, must be accommodated. A custom shoe with a "combination" last (narrow heel and wide forefoot) is usually required for both adequate toe space and good support by the heel counter. Additional heel inner lining can be added to standard shoes to achieve the same purpose.

Relief of pressure on the metatarsal heads can be accomplished by several means. Insertion of a *metatarsal pad* in the shoe just proximal to the distal metatarsal head may suffice to relieve the weight-bearing stress on that joint, or a metatarsal pad may be inserted in such a manner as to elevate all of the metatarsal heads where this is required.[141] A *heat-formed molded insert* of Plastazote may be fabricated quickly, by direct application of the warm material to the foot, providing a custom-fitted molded insole that can be very effective in relieving weight-bearing stresses. Although a Plastazote insole may need replacement every 3 to 6 months, it can be more economically fabricated than customized, carved sole reliefs of the "space" shoe, constructed on a mold prepared from a plaster cast of the foot.[316]

Many patients with metatarsalgia obtain benefit from an accurately positioned metatarsal bar, which consists of a firm, 1 to 1½ inch wide, ⅛ inch thick piece of leather placed horizontally on the external surface of the shoe just proximal to the wear line caused by the metatarsal weight-bearing surface.[152] These bars can be extended anteriorly and rounded to form a "rocker" surface, which may facilitate the toe-off phase of gait, but they have the disadvantage, particularly if the anterior surface is not tapered, of protruding sufficiently from the sole of the shoe to put the patient at the risk of tripping.[222]

The *"rocker" sole configuration,* with the arc extended beyond the MTP joints on an inflexible sole, offers a rigid supporting surface to *protect a painful arthritic first MTP joint* or a hallux rigidus during the toe-off phase of gait.[222] The latter problem can also be well managed by a removable metal insole with an extension to provide an internal rocker surface under the great toe.[152]

In the arthritic foot with talonavicular joint involvement or minimal pronation, stabilization and pain relief may be improved by the application of a 5.0 mm, medial heel wedge to a shoe with a rigid and well-fitted heel counter plus a compensating 3.0 to 4.0 mm. lateral sole wedge under the base of the fifth toe (to prevent the foot from sliding outward in the shoe).[142]

Although these suggestions are adequate to provide solutions to the vast majority of foot problems confronting the physician, the ideal solution to these problems requires, in addition to optimal rheumatological medical management, the thoughtful consideration of surgical alternatives and the collaboration of an orthotist, podiatrist, or professional prescription footwear provider capable of utilizing intelligently the wide variety of shoe and foot care adaptations that may need consideration for the solution of a given patient's problem.

SHOES—HEEL LIFT

Many patients with leg-length asymmetry, either congenital or as a consequence of hip, knee, or foot malalignment secondary to arthritis or trauma, may by the use of heel lifts obtain some relief from pain in the heel, leg, or back aggravated by mechanical stresses.

Because of the difficulty of identifying precise landmarks on the pelvis or upper femur (the anterior superior iliac spine and the superior margin of the greater trochanter are relatively diffuse landmarks), and the error introduced in measurement of the leg by relatively slight variations in position of the pelvis or thigh with a patient in bed, determinations of leg length with a tape measure are often imprecise. Radiographic determination of leg length has been shown to be precise, but is rarely needed in the assessment of functional leg length discrepancies in nonsurgical practice.[318]

A *practical method for measuring leg length* is the following: (1) The patient stands with his back to the examiner, who is seated on a low stool with his eyes approximately at the level of the iliac crests. (2) The patient places the back of both heels on a line and stands naturally with both feet parallel. (3) If either knee is bent, it is actively or passively extended as fully as possible. (4) The examiner then palpates the lateral superior margins of both iliac crests with his finger tips, holding his fingers extended and parallel to the floor. (5) Any discrepancy in the height of the iliac crests is interpreted as a functional leg length discrepancy, and boards of measured thickness (or books, magazines, or prescription pads) are placed under the short leg until the iliac crests are approximately level.

Correction of compensatory scoliosis, horizontal alignment of posterior superior iliac spines, gluteal folds, or popliteal creases, and elimination of soft tissue creases in the lateral trunk are all confirmatory of a functional leg length correction. In an adult of average height with a skeletal problem subject to aggravation during ambulation, a leg length discrepancy greater than 1.0 cm. should be corrected.

The rule of thumb is to make a shoe correction that compensates for approximately three-fourths of the leg length discrepancy. For geriatric patients the correction may be done in two or more stages one to three months apart to facilitate accommodation of skeletal structures to the changed alignment. If the correction is entirely built into a heel, the added stress on the forefoot may lead to metatarsalgia. If the heel on a shoe is raised over ½ inch, compensation by thickening the sole of that shoe (either on the insole or outside the shoe) is needed to balance the foot. A ¼ inch heel lift made of firm leather, cork, or neoprene can be placed inside the shoe or it can be placed under or sandwiched into the external heel.

A half-inch correction can be made either by placing the ¼ inch lift both inside and outside a heel or by adding ¼ inch to the heel of one shoe and removing ¼ inch from the heel of the opposite shoe. Correction of a ¾ inch leg length discrepancy can be achieved without the need to add any additional thickness to the sole of the shortened side by adding ¼ inch inside the heel of the shoe on the short side, ¼ inch outside the heel of the same shoe, and removing ¼ inch from the heel of the opposite shoe. (See Fig. 60.)

SPLINTING AND BRACING THE NECK

The most common indication for splinting or bracing the neck is to relieve local or referred pain as a consequence of cervical discogenic disease or strain. The basic objective here is to provide sufficient support to the neck to relieve inordinate movement and the chronic muscle tension or reflex muscle spasm that is a consequence of motion at a local discogenic, articular, or soft tissue source of irritation. Wearing a soft collar or a semirigid plastic splint, fitted to hold the neck in a comfortable neutral position or in slight flexion, usually gives symptomatic relief, although the actual role of the collar in providing that relief has been challenged.[116, 319, 320]

Studies on the immobilization efficiency of various types of cervical braces and collars have been performed on normal subjects, so that the basis for a decision as to what collar or brace is most efficient

TABLE 5–2.   Stabilizing Efficiency of Cervical Braces and Collars in Normal Subjects

	Soft Collar	Plastic Collar Submandibular	Plastic-collar-Brace Occipito-mental-sternal	4-poster Brace	Long 2-poster Brace	Halo
Comfort and convenience	excellent night and day, except in warm weather	good, cool, easily cleaned	good	fair	fair-poor, may need assistance to apply	poor
Vertebral Level						
C_1-Occiput						
Flex.-ext.	poor[1]	fair[2]	fair-good	fair-good	fair-good	excellent
Lateral bend	poor	fair	NS[3]	NS	good	excellent
Rotation	poor	fair	NS	good	good	excellent
C_2-C_1						
Flex.-ext.	poor	fair	fair-good	fair-good	excellent[5]	excellent
Lateral bend	poor	fair	NS	NS	good	excellent
Rotation	poor	poor	NS	fair	good	excellent
C_4-C_2						
Flex.-ext.	poor	fair	good[4]	good	excellent	excellent
Lateral bend	poor	fair	NS	good	good	excellent
Rotation	poor	fair	NS	good	good	excellent
T_1-C_4						
Flex.-ext.	poor	fair	fair	good-excellent	good	excellent
Lateral bend	poor	fair	NS	good	good	excellent
Rotation	poor	fair	NS	good	good	excellent
Features	foam rubber or felt covered with stockinette	should have ventilation holes and adjustment struts	The Philadelphia collar has molded chin and occipital supports made of Plastazote	anterior and posterior chest pieces secured with shoulder straps	fixed to chest with shoulder subaxillary straps	requires surgical scalp fixation

[1] Poor: 50 per cent restriction of motion
[2] Fair: 50 per cent to 20 per cent restriction of motion
[3] NS: not studied
[4] Good: 20 per cent to 5 per cent restriction of motion
[5] Excellent: 5 per cent or less residual motion

in a clinical setting is based on extrapolations from these studies and clinical experience, which includes experience relating to outcomes and to patients' tolerance of these devices.[116, 321-323] (See Tables 5-2 and 5-3.) Short of scalp fixation in a halo cast as a means of immobilizing the cervical spine, stabilization of the *lower* cervical spine can be accomplished by the use of a rigid cervical brace which incorporates a chin and occipital support plus shoulder and chest strap fixation to the chest, but even this extensive bracing does not reliably stabilize the upper cervical region.[321, 322, 324-327] (See Fig. 62.)

The 4-poster cervical brace and the Philadelphia collar are somewhat less cumbersome and almost as efficient in stabilizing the lower cervical spine as the braces that require chest fixation. [328] The *Philadelphia collar* tends to feel warm, but for severely involved patients is the most comfortable and usually the only effective cervical support that will be worn at night. (See Fig. 61.)

Rheumatoid arthritis typically involves both the middle cervical spine and the C_1–C_2 region. Symptoms may be caused by the local inflammatory process and, more importantly, can result from mechanical derangements associated with vertebral subluxations and spinal cord compression.[327] In one series of 130 patients with rheumatoid cervical spondylitis and subluxation, no protective advantage in terms of arresting the progress of subluxation was evident from the wearing of cervical collars.[325] These authors did not specify the kind of cervical splinting or bracing ("collars") used, but they did comment that 6 of

TABLE 5–3. Combined Functional and Comfort-Ranking for Cervical Collars and Braces

For general cervical pain relief, ease of application, day and night comfort, and economy, in the absence of a recent or progressive neurological deficit:
1. Soft collar
2. Plastic submandibular collar
3. Plastic collar-brace (Philadelphia type)

For high cervical instability with severe suboccipital pain:
1. Long 2-poster
2. Plastic collar-brace (Philadelphia type)
3. 4-poster

For high cervical instability with potentially catastrophic neurological deficit:
1. Halo fixation
2. Long 2-poster

For mid-cervical instability with severe pain or mild neurological deficit:
1. Long 2-poster
2. Plastic collar-brace (Philadelphia type)
3. 4-poster

For lower cervical instability with severe pain or mild neurological deficit:
1. 4-poster
2. Long 2-poster
3. Plastic collar-brace (Philadelphia type)

the 14 patients who wore their collars regularly continued to complain of pain, possibly attributable to a lack of neck support by the collars. Conversely, many of their patients chose not to wear their collars, apparently because the benefits did not offset the nuisance.[325]

It would appear that cervical splinting and bracing by any means provide insufficient stabilization to influence the progression of C_1–C_2 subluxations. Nonetheless, many patients with rheumatoid arthritis, as well as those with ankylosing spondylitis and discogenic disease, experience a temporary reduction of pain during exacerbations of cervical pain by wearing a soft collar (soft collars can be comfortably worn in bed) or a semirigid plastic (Philadelphia) collar that offers some degree of soft tissue support. These collars may provide some additional protection against the potentially catastrophic accidental hyperflexion of the unstable cervical spine that occurs with a flexion-extension injury or fall.[327, 329]

When a cervical collar or brace is prescribed, isometric exercises to the cervical flexor, extensor, and rotator muscle groups should be administered as soon as tolerated to minimize disuse atrophy. (See Fig. 47.) In the presence of weak cervical musculature secondary to myopathic or neuropathic disorders, the chin support must be adjusted and padded to minimize pressure.[330] For the patient with cervical arthritis who cannot tolerate a collar at night, a measure of cervical support may be obtained by the use of a small firm pillow made of multiple layers of dacron and crinoline (measuring 6 x 16 inches and 3 to 4 inches thick), designed to *support the neck in the supine position* and the *head in the side-lying position*. Another useful aid is a tubular-shaped contour *pillow* ("Cervipillo") sufficiently firm to support the head in the side-lying position and sufficiently compressible to minimize any flexion or extension of the neck in the supine or prone position, respectively.[331, 332]

SPINAL BRACING

The most common indication for the use of a spinal brace or corset is to relieve low back discomfort. The objectives of bracing are not only to relieve discomfort but to expedite remission of discomfort and prevent exacerbation of radiculopathy where root compression is a problem. In a classic study Norton and Brown demonstrated that *no brace was capable of effectively immobilizing the lumbosacral region.*[261] Not only is the lumbosacral spine not immobilized by bracing or corseting but, in fact, spinal motion may be increased at the segments adjacent to the upper and lower ends of the brace or corset.[333] It has been shown that axial rotation from a standing position can be reduced by a chairback brace, but this motion is minimally affected by the use of a corset and *both the corset and brace actually increase axial rotation during walking.*[262] The observation of continuing electromyographic activity in the abdominal and spinal muscles during ambulation in normal subjects wearing chairback braces and lumbosacral corsets provides additional indirect evidence of the failure of immobilization by these means.[334]

The instability of the vertebral column is so great that fixation of any brace to the pelvis is required for immobilization. For complete lumbar vertebral fixation this, in turn, necessitates extending a cast or brace below the pelvis to the thigh since firm pelvic fixation is nearly impossible to achieve.[261, 333, 335] In addition to reducing mobility of the spine, it is considered that spinal braces or corsets may serve to relieve inordinate loads on a compromised disk or otherwise stressed area of the spinal structures.[291, 336]

The abdominal compression component of spinal braces and corsets supplements or substitutes for the support of the abdominal musculature and may act in large part to relieve local stresses on the spinal column by creating a nearly rigid walled cylinder of soft tissue and viscera through which the stresses can be distributed.[291, 336, 337] This may explain in part the subjective relief of low back pain attributed to the wearing of narrow sacro-iliac "belts" or corsets.[333] Paradoxically, in a study of patients with low back pain, the strength of the abdominal muscles as measured by their maximum instantaneous tensions did not correlate with the presence or absence of persistent low back pain.[231] Whether any difference in this assessment would be achieved had the strength of the abdominal musculature been measured as a function of dynamic endurance rather than as static peak strength remains unanswered, but it would appear that muscular support or compression of the abdomen alone is not sufficient to relieve persistent painful low back stresses.

A survey of orthopedic surgeons served to underscore the lack of uniformity in their approach to back bracing but did reach something of a consensus in that bracing and corseting were generally prescribed for persistent low back pain, particularly when associated with spondylolysthesis, pseudoarthrosis, or as part of the management of postoperative treatment.[335] In that study external supports were generally not prescribed for "acute strain, the postoperative disk, or for a person with obesity and pain."[335] Again, referring to the above study, opinion was equally divided as to whether a brace or corset would be prescribed for any particular problem, but when a brace was prescribed the chairback model was the one usually selected.[335]

GENERAL CONSIDERATIONS IN CORSET FITTING

When fitted in the standing position, the corset or brace should extend well over the buttock, approaching the horizontal gluteal fold posteriorly. Lacing, snaps, or Velcro closures should create a snug fit.

(See Figs. 63 and 64.) The *corset is often most easily applied when the patient is in bed by rolling from side-lying* onto the corset in a supine position or, secondarily, by *standing and leaning with the low back against a wall* for support while cinching the corset.

When the patient is seated the corset should permit sufficient freedom of movement at the groin so that there is no compression of soft tissue and, except for patients with hypersensitivity of the rib cage, should extend to include the lower rib margins laterally, and to 5.0 cm below the scapular tips posteriorly. Corsets that are provided with pliable stays to assist in maintaining corset form and fit may sometimes require contoured steel stays to increase rigidity and provide a better purchase for counterpressure.[333]

SUMMARY — LOW
BACK BRACING AND CORSETING

A lumbosacral corset or low back brace apparently serves primarily to provide some restriction or inhibition of spinal movement and may additionally function to redistribute load stresses by abdominal compression. The author uses a lumbosacral *corset* to provide pain relief and facilitate earlier return to functional activities for the patient with slowly subsiding acute low back pain, with or without radiculopathy, and for many patients with chronic low back pain as well. An occasional male who engages in hard physical work prefers a chairback brace to a corset. Regular exercise to maintain mobility of the lumbar and gluteal musculature and strength of the abdominal and gluteal musculature is prescribed for virtually all patients for whom a corset or brace is provided.[338]

The most common indication for *thoracolumbar bracing* arises in the patient with osteoporosis and compression fracture. The use of a thoracolumbar corset extending over the scapulae, with shoulder straps to maintain position, is often of considerable help in obtaining pain relief in these cases.[333] (See Fig. 65.) A thoracolumbar, or Taylor, brace, because of its greater rigidity, might be assumed to have advantages over a corset in providing relief for discomfort associated with vertebral body compression fractures, or for pain associated with severe dorsal kyphosis, epiphysitis, or ankylosing spondylitis. The Taylor brace is, however, only minimally effective as a means of stabilizing the dorsal spine, and its chief advantage over a corset is in providing better ventilation.[333] In patients with severe osteoporosis, multiple compression fractures, or tumor, such as multiple myeloma or metastatic cancer, the use of a body jacket made from a plaster cast mold may be required for stability and relief.[333]

Patients with *ankylosing spondylitis* usually obtain sufficient relief from medication to comply with posture and exercise regimens so that bracing or corseting for pain relief is rarely prescribed. Further, there is no convincing evidence that braces prevent spinal deformity in ankylosing spondylitis. The application of bracing to correct scoliotic deformities is a highly specialized process in which a brace utilizing pelvic and cervical fixation with adjustable spinal curvature correcting pads is employed.[338, 339]

SELECTED READINGS BY TOPICS

(See also complete Bibliography on page 213.)

General Orthotic Considerations

143. American Rheumatism Association, Arthritis and Rheumatism Foundation and National Institute of Arthritis and Metabolic Diseases: Chapter 3. Evaluation of Splinting. Criteria for and evaluation of orthopedic measures in the management of deformities of rheumatoid arthritis. Arthritis Rheum., 7, (5), Part 2:585, 1964.
259. Rizzo, F., Hamilton, B. B., Keagy, R. D.: Orthotics research evaluation framework. Arch. Phys. Med. Rehabil., 56:304, Jul. 1975.
265. Rotstein, J.: Use of splints in conservative management of acutely inflamed joints in rheumatoid arthritis. Arch. Phys. Med., 46:198, Feb. 1965.
270. Harris, R.: "Chapter 14. Plaster splints for rheumatoid arthritis," in S. Licht, H. Kamenetz, eds., Orthotics Etcetera. New Haven: E. Licht, 1966. Pp. 336–346.

Hand Orthoses

150. Flatt, A. E.: "Chapter 3. Nonoperative treatment," in A. E. Flatt, ed., The Care of the Rheumatoid Hand. 3rd Ed. St. Louis. C. V. Mosby Co., 1974. P. 33.
258. Malick, M. H.: Manual on Dynamic Hand Splinting with Thermoplastic Materials. Pittsburgh, Pa.: Harmarville Rehabilitation Center, 1974.
281. Bunnell, S.: Surgery of the Hand. 3rd Ed. Philadelphia: J. B. Lippincott Co., 1956. Pp. 539, 552–554.
285. Malick, M. H.: Manual on Static Hand Splinting. Vol. 1. Pittsburgh, Pa.: Harmarville Rehabilitation Center, 1972. Pp. 32, 45, 76, 93.
287. Bennett, R. L.: "Wrist and hand slip-on splints," in S. Licht, ed., Arthritis and Physical Medicine. Baltimore: Waverly Press, 1969. P. 482.
289. Bennett, R. L.: Orthotic devices to prevent deformities of the hand in rheumatoid arthritis. Arthritis Rheum., 8:1006, Oct. 1965.
298. Bunnell, S.: Surgery of the Hand. 5th Ed. Revised by Boyes, J. H. Philadelphia: J. B. Lippincott Co., 1970. Pp. 171-176.
301. Long, C.: "Chapter 10. Upper limb bracing," in S. Licht, H. Kamenetz, eds., Orthotics Etcetera. New Haven: E. Licht, 1966. P. 152.

Neck Orthoses

319. Brewerton, D. A., et al.: Pain in the neck and arm: a multicentre trial of the effects of physiotherapy. Br. Med. J., 1:253, 1966.
322. Johnson, R. M., et al.: Functional evaluation of cervical collars and braces. Abstract, American Congress of Rehabilitation Medicine, 53rd Annual Session, San Diego, November 11, 1976.
323. Fisher, S. V., et al.: Cervical orthoses effect on cervical spine motion: Roentgenographic and gonimetric method of study. Arch. Phys. Med. Rehabil, 58:109, Mar. 1977.
325. Smith, P. H., Sharp, J., Kellgren, J. A.: Natural history of rheumatoid cervical subluxations. Ann. Rheum. Dis., 31:222, May 1972.
326. Conlon, P. W., Isdale, I. C., Rose, B. S.: Rheumatoid arthritis of the cervical spine. An analysis of 333 cases. Ann. Rheum. Dis., 25:120, Mar. 1966.

Back Orthoses

261. Norton, P. L., Brown, T.: The immobilizing efficiency of back braces. J. Bone Joint Surg., 39A (1):111, 1957.

262. Lumsden, R. M., Morris, J. M.: An in vivo study of axial rotation and immobilization at the lumbosacral joint. J. Bone Joint Surg., *50A:* 1591, Dec. 1968.

Knee Orthoses

264. Lehmann, J. F., Warren, C. G.: Restraining forces in various designs of knee ankle orthoses: their placement and effect on the anatomical knee joint. Arch. Phys. Med. Rehabil., *57*:430, Sept. 1976.
272. Jayson, M. I., Dixon, A. S.: Intra-articular pressure in rheumatoid arthritis of the knee. 3. Pressure changes during joint use. Ann. Rheum. Dis. *29*:401, July 1970.
273. DeAndrade, J. R., Grant, C., Dixon, A. S.: Joint distension and reflex muscle inhibition in the knee. J. Bone Joint Surg., *47A*:313, Mar. 1965.
305. Deaver, G. G.: "Chapter 11. Lower limb bracing" *in* S. Licht, H. Kamenetz, eds., *Orthotics Etcetera.* New Haven: E. Licht, 1966. Pp. 249, 266.
307. Lehneis, H. R., Bergofsky, E., Frisina, W.: Energy expenditure with advanced lower limb orthoses and with conventional braces. Arch. Phys. Med. Rehabil, *57*:20, Jan. 1976.
311. Smith, E. M., Juvinall, R. C., Corell, E. B., et al.: Bracing the unstable arthritic knee. Arch. Phys. Med. Rehabil., *51*:22, Jan. 1970.

Foot Orthoses

222. Cailliet, R.: *Foot and Ankle Pain.* Philadelphia: F. A. Davis Company, 1968. Pp. 89–110.
313. Swezey, R. L.: Below-knee weight-bearing brace for the arthritic foot. Arch. Phys. Med. Rehabil., *56*:176, Apr. 1975.
315. Campbell, J. W., Inman, V. T.: Treatment of plantar fasciitis and calcaneal spurs with the UC-BL shoe insert. Clin. Orthop., *103*:57, 1974.
316. Zamosky, I., Licht, S.: "Chapter 18. Shoes and their modification," *in* S. Licht, H. Kamenetz, eds., *Orthotics Etcetera.* New Haven: E. Licht, 1966. P. 403.

Chapter 6

MOBILITY AND MOVEMENT BARRIERS

Canes, Crutches, Wheelchairs,
Automobiles, and Architectural
Barriers

Mobility problems commence at any point of departure, whether it be from a bed, toilet, chair or couch, or standing surface. *In order to become mobile,* the person with a physical disability *must first be able to transfer* from a lying position to a sitting position or from a sitting position to a standing position and ultimately to reverse the process. *Furnishings should be designed* to create optimal comfort, prevent deformity, and *facilitate transfer.*

Low chairs or couches, soft cushions, or sagging and soft mattresses create difficulties for a patient who must first move himself into a position from which he can then transfer.[235] The yielding mattress or seat cushion offers no support over which the patient can slide and he must strain muscles and joints in order to compensate for the yielding and fluctuating surface over which he has to move to change position. (See Figs. 40 to 42). Further, if the seat, couch, or bed is too close to the floor, the hips and knees are markedly flexed and stressed while the weight of the body is lifted against gravity on standing.

A proper seat should be firmly padded and positioned at a height such that when the patient sits his feet are comfortably supported on the ground or placed on a low stool. This serves to minimize excessive pressure on the posterior thigh soft tissue and neuromuscular structures caused by dangling feet, as well as to minimize the shortening of the Achilles tendon that occurs with the feet hanging in plantar flexion. With the hips flexed to an angle of approximately 90 degrees, or even slightly greater than 90 degrees, the patient does not have to

127

struggle to raise his center of gravity up to the level of the knees, and so can much more readily arise. (See Fig. 51.)

Important *devices to facilitate transfer are chair arms, railings, bed side-rails, and chairs designed so that a patient can place his feet beneath him* when transferring from a seated to a standing position.[238, 239] Other furnishings that may enhance mobility, circumvent unnecessary or dangerous mobility (e.g., getting up for toileting at night), or obviate the problems of excessive prolonged immobility include the following: bedboards sufficient to prevent both side-to-side and head-to-toe sagging in the mattress; raised toilet seats with adjacent hand rails or grab bars; shower seats and grab bars; bathtub benches and railings; and even bedside commodes or adapted bedpans.[238, 239, 310] *Optimal mobility is often dependent on the instruction* of the family and nursing personnel in *specific techniques* for the safe transfer of the patient from a bed to a wheelchair or to a toilet or bath.[238, 239, 251, 340-342]

GAIT

In ambulation patients can be roughly categorized as: (1) nonambulatory, (2) household ambulator, (3) community ambulator, and (4) normal. Normal gait is an extremely efficient, low-energy-consuming activity.[343-345] Modifications of gait as a result of weakness, pain, and joint deformity and instability create difficulty on ambulation on a horizontal surface and even greater difficulty on an irregular surface and on ascending or descending an incline, with or without steps. The greater the instability of gait, the greater the energy required to ambulate, with resultant accentuation of fatigue, increased weakness, and risk of falling, or exhaustion of cardiorespiratory reserve in patients with cardiopulmonary problems.[343, 345, 346]

A major requisite for an efficient gait is free and full motion of joints. Any joint contracture will perforce lead to alterations of gait and stress on the compensating articular and periarticular structures. Proper footwear, correction of leg length discrepancies, utilization of appropriate bracing (see previous discussions of footwear, leg length and bracing), and most often the use of an ambulation assistive device, namely, cane, crutch, walker, railing, and, during training, parallel bars, can improve the efficiency of gait.[345-347]

CANE AND CRUTCH FITTING

It is unfortunate that our society has stigmatized the cane as a sign of weakness, for there is probably no assistive device more efficiently designed for its task. Walter Blount, in a classic article entitled "Don't Throw Away the Cane," has eloquently put forth not only the importance of the cane, but the rationale for its proper use.[348] The cane is not the only ambulation assistive device, nor is a cane one standard item, for it must be properly fitted in terms of length, weight, and grip configuration in order to function effectively for the arthritic patient.

For *adjusting the hand grip* position or for measuring the length of a cane or crutch, the patient should stand with his feet comfortably planted and his elbow flexed at a 15 to 30 degree angle. In that position, the tip of the cane or crutch (covered with a skid-proof crutch tip) should reach a point approximately 8 inches lateral to the tip of the toes. The position of the hand grip is not arbitrary. It is determined by the most comfortable elbow angle required for stability at mid-stance that will also allow for adequate reach during the swing phase of gait. Appropriate modifications are necessary in cases with elbow or wrist contractures.

The axillary pad of the standard crutch should touch the lateral chest wall at a point two finger breadths below the anterior axillary fold. The clearance in the axilla is designed to prevent compression on the axillary vessels and brachial plexus due to leaning on the crutch. A single cane or crutch is carried in the hand opposite the affected lower extremity joint in order to permit the most efficient gait with the least stress on the upper extremity joints through which weight-bearing forces are transmitted via the cane.[239, 348]

For the arthritic patient with multiple joint involvement there are available a variety of modifications of crutches and canes and walkers designed to accommodate fixed contractures, painful upper extremity joints, weakness of hand grasp, and instability of both upper and lower extremity joints.[238, 239] Notable among these are the platform forearm support modifications for crutches or walkers that shift weight bearing from the arthritic hand and wrist or extended elbow joints to the forearm and flexed elbow. (See Fig. 66.) Excellent references on gait training provide illustrated examples of techniques to teach ambulation in a variety of disabilities and with various assistive devices.[142, 239, 349, 350]

Many severely involved arthritic patients are capable of limited ambulation, but practical ambulation, even in the household, is not feasible for some. Useful mobility in these cases requires the utilization of a *wheelchair*. The prescription of a wheelchair demands a great deal of sophistication lest an expensive but totally inappropriate piece of equipment be provided to a patient already sufficiently encumbered by a physical handicap and desperately needing a well-designed, well-functioning mobility resource.

There are a number of wheelchair manufacturers, and each manufacturer has several models that range in quality and variety of optional features in a manner reminiscent of the automotive industry. The wheelchair should literally be fitted to the patient, with due consideration given to the height, width, and depth of the seat; the height and design of the arm rests, or indeed whether or not arm rests should be provided; the height of the back (and whether or not it should be zippered to facilitate certain types of transfers); reclining feature; head-rest features; elevating and removable foot rests; durability of construction, dependent on the weight of the user and the surfaces over which the chair will be operating. In addition, rim handholds, brake positions, front wheel caster size, and even color must be considered.

Particular attention must be given to the wheelchair's width. The average adult wheelchair measures 24½ inches from hub to hub and varies with the width of the seat. This width can be a crucial factor in precluding access of a wheelchair patient to a bathroom because many bathroom doors cannot be opened sufficiently to permit wheelchair entrance. Provision of wheelchairs whose axles can be narrowed or "junior" size chairs, for patients who can be accommodated in them, may solve an otherwise difficult problem. Additional accessories and options include seat cushions designed to minimize the threat of decubitus ulceration and power options.

Detailed descriptions of wheelchair configurations and the appropriate considerations in determining the components of a wheelchair prescription can be found in several excellent references as well as obtained from the wheelchair manufacturers themselves.[237, 239, 351-354] As with all mechanical equipment, the availability and quality of service for wheelchairs, all other things being equal, should be an overriding consideration in the final selection of the item to be purchased. If wheelchairs are to be used for only short periods of time, many of these considerations may be overlooked, but if the patient is to use the wheelchair as a significant long-term mobility resource, then appropriate consultation with a knowledgeable therapist should be obtained prior to making the not insignificant investment in the purchase of a wheelchair.

TRANSPORTATION

An essential component of mobility for almost all of us is the automobile. Any disturbance of joint function, except perhaps in the temporomandibular joints, may create problems for the automobile driver. Car door access, seat height, and back support, visibility, doorknobs, starter keys, steering ease, dimmer switches, braking, ease of seat adjustment, and access to controls all pose potential problems to the patients with arthritis who must drive. A variety of automobile adaptations are now available to facilitate access to and control of automobiles by handicapped persons.[238, 355, 356] Special programs developed for assessing a driver's capability and adaptability to automobile modifications in actual driving conditions can provide an essential dimension to the potentially mobile person who is otherwise unable to operate a standard vehicle independently.[357-360]

Considerations relating to public transportation and conveyances, including air travel, are further discussed in Chapter 8 under *Recreational Facilities*.

In order for mobility to be entirely functional one has to have access to his final destination. To find the parking lot full after a trip across town is exasperating to anyone, but to someone with significant impairment in ambulation or who needs a wheelchair, this inconvenience can reach a level of total frustration. The parking lot analogy can be carried further to curbs that cannot be mounted by wheelchair patients or many crutch and cane walkers, inaccessible steps, narrow doors, drinking fountains that are placed too high for patients confined to wheelchairs, lavatory facilities that cannot be entered or used by persons confined to wheelchairs, doorknobs that cannot be turned, faucets that cannot be turned on, inaccessible light switches, unreachable public telephones, slippery floors, and restaurant booths and cafeteria lines that cannot be negotiated. To complete a full circle of architectural barriers (without mentioning many other possible considerations) one can point out the need for close proximity of parking space to the final destination and the 12 foot minimum space width needed to permit patients with wheelchairs or on braces or crutches to get in and out of a car on a level surface.[31, 44, 238, 239, 361, 362]

SELECTED READINGS BY TOPICS

(See also complete Bibliography on page 213.)

Furniture and Transfers

44. Kliment, S. A.: *Into the Mainstream — A Syllabus for a Barrier-Free Environment.* U.S. Department of Health, Education and Welfare, Rehabilitation Services Administration. The American Institutes of Architects, Social and Rehabilitation Services, 1975. P. 26.

238. May, E. E., Waggoner, N. R., Hotte, E. B.: *Independent Living for the Handicapped and the Elderly.* Boston: Houghton Mifflin Company, 1974. Pp. 120, 251.

239. Lowman, E. W., Klinger, J. L.: *Aids to Independent Living: Self-Help for the Handicapped.* New York: McGraw-Hill, Inc. 1969.

340. *Rehabilitative Nursing Techniques — 1: Bed Positioning and Transfer Procedures for the Hemiplegic.* Minneapolis, Minn.: Kenny Rehabilitation Institute, 1964.

341. Laging, B.: Furniture design for the elderly. Rehab. Lit., *27*:130, May 1966.

Gait

349. Sorenson, L., Ulrich, P. G.: *Ambulation: A Manual for Nurses.* Minneapolis, Minnesota: American Rehabilitation Foundation, 1966.

350. Cicenia, E. F., Hoberman, M.: Crutch management drills. Modern Medicine, *26* (9):86, 1958.

Wheelchairs

351. Kamenetz, H. L.: "Chapter 21. Wheelchairs," *in* S. Licht, H. L. Kamenetz, eds., *Orthotics Etcetera.* New Haven: E. Licht, 1966. P. 473.

Handicapped Drivers

355. American Automobile Association: *Vehicle Controls for Disabled Persons.* Washington, D.C., 1973.
356. The Gazette: *Vans, busses, hydraulic lifts, and public transportation.* St. Louis, Missouri: Rehabilitation Gazette, 1973.
358. "Driver Education for the Handicapped." Des Moines Public School District and Younker Memorial Rehabilitation Center in cooperation with the National Highway Traffic Safety Administration and the Department of Public Instruction. n.d.

Architectural Barriers

361. Kira, A.: Housing needs of the aged with a guide to functional planning for the elderly and handicapped. Rehab. Lit., *21*:370, Dec. 1960.
362. Ramsey, C. G., Sleeper, H. R.: *Architectural Graphic Standards.* 6th Ed. New York: John Wiley & Sons, Inc., 1970. Pp. 4–5.

Chapter 7

THERAPEUTIC MODALITIES FOR PAIN RELIEF

Superficial Heat and Cold, Diathermy, Ultrasound, Hydrotherapy, Traction Massage and Manipulation, Vapo-coolant Spray and Local Injection Therapy, Transcutaneous Stimulation, Biofeedback, Acupuncture, Electrical Stimulation

Physical therapy traditionally stems from the utilization of physical measures, including literally earth, air, fire, and water, and later adding various segments of the electromagnetic spectrum as they were discovered (most notably X rays); in current practice it utilizes a variety of agents capable of producing physical stimuli. Various therapeutic modalities have had their vogue (bathing in water was once a radical and chic therapy), and their therapeutic effectiveness has been attributed to that which was capable of measurement (temperature, voltage, magnetic field effect) or that could be sold in the currency of speculation and "verified" by summation of anecdotal reports.[363] The chief therapeutic modalities in current use for the treatment of rheumatic disorders are the long-used therapies of superficial heating or cooling (fire and water) and deep heating.

PLACEBO PHENOMENON

Any discussion of the use of therapeutic modalities for pain relief must be couched in phrases that pay due respect to what is known and, more importantly, to what is not known about the mechanism of action of these modalities and (perhaps of greater import) to the impact of placebo phenomena on the therapeutic process. The enormous public expenditures on quack arthritic cures bear not so silent testimony to the therapeutic potency of placebos.

In all fairness to the difficulties the sophisticated clinician-therapist has in attempting to justify rationally the use of various therapeutic modalities and procedures in the treatment of painful musculoskeletal conditions, it should be pointed out, for example, that the rationale for making a choice among a variety of nonsteroidal anti-inflammatory drugs for any given patient is also open to searching questions.[364-366] Even the effect of intra-articular steroid injections in patients with rheumatoid arthritis and osteoarthritis has been shown to be difficult to distinguish from that of placebo injections.[367, 368]

If such factors as the degree of anxiety the patient has about his illness or whether his pill is red or white, let alone the attitude of the therapist, influence the apparent efficacy of a treatment, then it is not surprising that there is so little sound evidence upon which to judge the value of the various therapeutic procedures and modalities used in arthritis management.[369-372] There is, in fact, considerable evidence to document the enormous impact of placebo effects on responses to the use of therapeutic modalities, and any statement regarding the effectiveness of a modality on pain relief or improvement in performance of a functional task must be made with full appreciation of the impact of the placebo phenomenon.[366, 373-375]

SUPERFICIAL HEATING MODALITIES

Superficial heating modalities utilize infrared radiation by conduction from various sources of heat, including light bulbs, fireplaces and infrared irradiators, as well as infrared heating by contact with warm objects such as heating pads, moistened warm towels, hot packs, warm water, paraffin, and, less commonly, mud baths, warm sand and warm moist air (sauna). Like light, infrared energy is dissipated from its source in accordance with the inverse square law. Convective heating occurs when energy is transferred from a heat source via a liquid in motion, e.g., an agitated warm water bath. Conductive heating occurs on direct contact with a heat source and is a function of the specific heat of that source.[376] The high temperatures of paraffin in oil (52.0° C.) are well tolerated because paraffin transfers less heat than water (the specific heat of paraffin is only 0.5 while that of water is 1.0).[376]

From the physiological standpoint, a few facts that seem relevant to the efficacy of superficial heating in articular disorders can be stated. First, it can be demonstrated that *the threshold for pain can be raised in both man and animals by superficial or deep heating*.[377-380] Second, the skin penetration of superficial (infrared) heating is rarely more than a few millimeters in depth, and hence direct penetration into joints is the exception.[381-383] Third, changes in superficial as well as intra-articular circulation have been demonstrated as a consequence of superficial heating. An increase in joint circulation in osteoarthritis but a decrease in rheumatoid arthritis, as measured by radioactive sodium clearance from the heated joint, has been reported.[384, 385]

Superficial heating of extensive areas of body surface (warm tub at temperature of 37° C or greater) can cause an elevation in the total body temperature with a concurrent increase in metabolic demands.[386, 387] Peripheral vasodilatory effects may result in circulatory insufficiency and consequent local tissue ischemia, coronary artery or cerebrovascular ischemia, or in burns when peripheral blood flow is insufficient to conductively remove heat locally.[388, 389] The *demonstrable increases of superficial circulation* have been used as objective measures of the effect of superficial heating, but their *relevance to pain relief and muscle relaxation has not been determined*.[387]

COOLING MODALITIES

It is ironic that cold applications, which have been shown to reduce both skin and muscle temperature and have long been considered to be aggravating factors in arthritic and musculoskeletal painful disorders, are also useful in therapy.[390, 391] Superficial cooling has been demonstrated to reduce muscle spindle activity and to raise the threshold for pain.[390, 392] It has been shown in experimental animals that superficial cooling over joints with urate crystal–induced synovitis reduced xenon clearance and synovial fluid leukocytosis, while the converse was true for joint heating. Chronic synovitis from repeated crystal injections was not altered by heat or cold in this study.[393] The abrupt application of cold, however, causes discomfort and potentially stressful cardiovascular responses, which can be minimized by the initial interposition of a warm towel on which the cold compress is then placed.[376, 394] Contraindications to cold therapy include Raynaud's phenomenon, cold hypersensitivity, cryoglobulinemia, and paroxysmal cold hemoglobinuria.[376, 394]

The efficacy of specific superficial heating and cooling measures (including dry heat, moist heat, paraffin, ice packs, and ice massage) in terms of relief of pain or reduction in inflammation in either rheumatoid arthritis or osteoarthritis has not been established.[392, 394-399, 400] Moist heat is reported to be capable of raising subcutaneous temperature to a greater extent than dry heat, and although this coincides with the general impression that moist heat is preferable for relieving articular pain, the significance of this observation in terms of mechanisms of pain relief or alteration of inflammatory processes in joint disease has not been determined.[383, 401] Decisions about the use of superficial heat or cold for pain relief must, therefore, be made arbitrarily. They are based on *empirical observations that pain relief for acute inflammatory and traumatic states is best achieved by cold compresses, while subacute to chronic inflammation is best relieved by superficial heat.*[376, 400, 402-405] *In the presence of inflammatory articular disease, moist heat is generally more comforting than dry heat,* regardless of whether the mode of application is through the use of a hot pack or administered as hydrotherapy in a tub, shower, or pool. The prevention of chilling by avoidance of exposure to dampness, cold, and drafts, and by the use of insulating clothing to retain body heat, seems to help prevent exacerbations of chronic articular and periarticular disorders.

DIATHERMY

Deep heating, or diathermy (which means "heating through"), is effected by the use of short wave (11.0 meters at 27.33 MHz) or microwave (12.2 cm. at 2456 MHz) electromagnetic irradiations, or by the conversion to heat of high-frequency sound waves (approximately 1.0 MHz) in body tissues.[406] Greater penetration of tissues can be achieved by the use of the various deep heating modalities as compared with superficial heating, but only ultrasound has the capability of heating deeply situated articular structures such as the hip joint.[406-409] Like infrared, ultrasound has been shown to raise the pain threshold when applied over a peripheral nerve in normal human subjects.[378, 380] Circulatory changes occurring during diathermy are attributable largely to heat effects.[410, 411] Microwave diathermy has also been shown to cause in vitro alterations of human gamma globulin, independent of temperature effects.[412]

Deep heating has been demonstrated to affect the visco-elastic properties of collagen and increase the "creep" (plastic stretch) of ligamentous structures placed under tension.[413-416] A possible clinical application of this phenomenon may be enhanced efficacy of stretching therapies; however, the superiority of deep heating used expressly for this purpose over superficial heating for pain relief and muscle relaxation prior to or during stretching has not been substantiated.[416, 417]

The role of *ultrasound* as a deep heating modality is well established in clinical usage. The demonstration of its ability to heat deep structures suggests that ultrasound may have certain specific applications.[407-409, 417, 418] The utilization of ultrasound versus other diathermies in a variety of painful disorders is biased toward the selection of ultrasound in focal neuritic or periarthritic painful conditions. This choice is based on customary use and "conventional wisdom" but cannot be substantiated by any definitive study. It should be borne in mind, however, that this empirical approach is of necessity just as widely accepted in many other common therapeutic decisions where either insufficient investigation or a lack of sensitive measurements leaves the clinician with no other alternative.

Problems realting to ultrasound and other forms of diathermy generally include the possibility of burning patients who have poor circulation, impaired sensation, or metal implants and of aggravating bleeding diatheses and spreading malignant tumors.[419, 420] Care must be taken to avoid thermal injury as a consequence of electromagnetic waves (microwave and shortwave diathermy), which are concentrated by bone in fluid-filled cavities or by surface moisture.[421, 422] Testicular and lenticular damage as a consequence of heat generated by the absorption of electromagnetic radiation and the concentration of electromagnetic irradiation by metallic implants leading to tissue destruction have been documented.[406, 421-427] Ultrasound, by its great penetration, may cause damage to the spinal cord in the postlaminectomy patient.[419] Although malignant tumors and bleeding diatheses are considered contraindications to the use of deep heating modalities, evidence for this is anecdotal.[419, 420] Currently, the adjunctive role of deep heating in cancer therapy is being studied.[428-430]

Both short wave and microwave are administered in 20 to 30 minute treatments once or twice daily or three times weekly. *Short wave diathermy* is applied by either capacitive or inductive applicators and must be tuned to the individual patient.[413, 431] *Microwaves* are directed by an antenna and also require adjustment of dosage to individual tolerance.[413]

Both short wave and microwave diathermy are contraindicated in patients with cardiac pacemakers.[427] All commercial diathermy devices are standardized but must receive periodic calibration to ensure proper function.[419, 432, 433] There is no convincing evidence that pulsed diathermy (or ultrasound) has any advantage over continuous energy inputs, as the effects are due to the total energy delivered.[406, 425] *Ultrasound* has the advantage that it is reflected rather than concentrated by metal and therefore can be used in the presence of metallic implants; however, its safety when used over metal prosthetic implants embedded in methylmethacrylate has not been established.[419, 434] Ultrasound transmission requires the use of a coupling agent (water or mineral oil) to prevent dampening of sound waves in air.[419] The ultrasound applicator must be kept in constant motion by the therapist in order to minimize excessive focal heating, or the cavitation phenomenon that may result from highly focused ultrasound irradiation.[419] Ultrasound is administered in doses of from 0.5 to 3.0 watts/cm.^{2} for from 3 to 15 minutes, depending on tolerance and the depth and size of the area treated.

SUMMARY OF HEATING AND
COOLING MODALITIES

Diathermy administered by electromagnetic or ultrasound instrumentation can be shown to produce deep heating, with the greatest depth achievable by ultrasound. Thus far no clear demonstration has been made of any advantage for deep heating on pain relief, but conventional wisdom would have it that in chronic painful disorders deep heating may be more effective than superficial cold or heat.[418, 435] Ultrasound may be of particular value in focal neuralgic or periarticular painful conditions.[419] The usual duration of treatment with heating or cooling modalities is 20 to 30 minutes. With mild heating or cooling, or when local areas are treated, treatments may be extended to one hour. Ultrasound is the exception, with treatment usually given for 5 to 15 minutes.

Further study to define the precise role of these modalities and to distinguish their specific effects and efficacy when compared with placebos is clearly indicated. The danger of thermal injury with any heat modality is increased in the presence of poor circulation, sedation, or sensory impairment. This is particularly true of the use of diathermy because the minimal heating of superficial tissues that occurs creates little thermal sensation, and excessive heating may be detected too late to prevent thermal injury.[388, 402] The evidence that collagenases in rheumatoid synovia show increased activity in the presence of temperature elevation raises serious questions about the efficacy of vigorous heating in the presence of inflammatory arthritic processes.[436, 437] In rheumatic disease problems efforts to demonstrate advantages for diathermy (including ultrasound) over superficial heat or cold methodologies have not proved successful.[392, 396, 406, 417, 435, 438, 439]

HYDROTHERAPY OPTIONS

Hydrotherapy has long been used for providing both heat and the buoyancy of water for relief of painful articular disorders. A variety of methods include the use of arm or leg basins, with or without water agitators (whirlpools), tubs and specially designed therapeutic tanks (Hubbard tank), therapeutic pools, as well as conventional recreational swimming pools.[159, 440, 441] The selection of the basin or tub depends on the specific joints involved, with a large tank or pool being particularly desirable for patients with multiple joint or lower extremity large joint involvement. The therapeutic and recreational pools not only provide a medium for total body immersion and heat transference but can also be utilized effectively for specific therapeutic exercise, for swimming as a general conditioning exercise, and for graduated ambulation training facilitated by superficial heating and the support to painful or weakened structures provided by the buoyancy of water.[442, 443]

The concerns regarding elevation of body temperature either locally or generally with any heating modality obviously apply in the use of hydrotherapy. The enervating and relaxing consequences of *total emergence in warm water* are compounded by peripheral vasodilation. In a healthy person this can result in a sensation of weakness; in a patient whose circulatory reserve is compromised, it may result in collapse and injury (even after leaving the pool), or in myocardial or cerebral ischemia.

Generalized peripheral vasodilation can be produced by slowly increasing the water temperature from 37° C to 45° C for a 20 minute immersion of an arm or foot, or as a sitz bath.[159, 441] Exposure of small areas of the skin in water at 46° C cannot be tolerated for more than a few minutes. For total body immersion, a tank, tub or pool is usually maintained at 32 to 38° C, at which temperatures the patient feels comfortably warm and a generalized vasodilation takes place.[159, 440, 441] The duration of total immersion should not exceed five minutes initially in debilitated patients, and the optimal duration of treatment is usually 20 to 30 minutes. The addition of controlled agitation of the water by a whirlpool mechanism provides a gentle to brisk massaging sensation which is usually comforting to the arthritic patient.[441] Because the expense of individual tank therapy is usually great, this modality should be carefully prescribed and promptly terminated when goals are achieved or no progress is being made. This is often difficult because patients enjoy the tank or pool therapy and are usually reluctant to give it up if they are not responsible for meeting its expense.

TRACTION

The role of traction in relieving pain or overcoming flexion contractures in the arthritic knee and hip is well established.[111, 142-145, 148, 149] Specific methods for the application of knee traction in flexion contractures are well described by Stein et al.[144] (See Fig. 28.) More controversial is the role of traction as a force system applied to the body along its length in an effort to separate vertebral or spinal structures. It is common knowledge that stretching provides a measure of relief when one feels stiffness or tightness in his muscles after exercise or experiences a cramp from whatever cause.

A basic question with regard to traction as it is applied to the cervical and lumbar spine is not whether any benefits claimed can be attributed to a nonspecific musculoskeletal passive stretching phenomenon but whether there is a more specific effect on skeletal structures. This might occur as a consequence of distraction of intervertebral disk spaces or facet joints that could cause disk material to move away either from the sensitive periphery of the annulus or from nerve root contact, or by traction facilitated realignment of displaced (subluxated) facet joints.[444]

With regard to *traction on the lumbar spine,* it has become apparent that unless frictional forces are eliminated by the use of a specially designed split-sliding table, or by forces sufficient to overcome the coefficient of the friction of a body in a bed (approximately 0.5), traction as customarily applied to the pelvis or legs is not sufficient to cause intradiscal and facet joint separation.[232, 445-451] Studies in normal subjects utilizing either a horizontal split-table with countertraction on the chest, or a vertical distraction device employing forces up to 300 pounds, have demonstrated elongation of the spine and evidence of up to 2.2 mm. of widening of the L_4–L_5 and L_5–S_1 intervertebral joint spaces.[452, 453] In a preliminary trial on ten patients with lumbar discogenic disease and on seven patients with an acute protruded intervertebral disk syndrome, the use of split-table traction (a two-piece table constructed to permit the portion supporting the patient's legs and pelvis to slide in order to eliminate friction) was credited for at least partial subjective benefit in all patients.[453]

Failure of this method of traction, however, and exacerbation of root pain has been attributed to downward traction of a lumbar or sacral root over an extruded disk fragment.[448, 454] Although separation of discal spaces has been demonstrated in at least two studies on normal young subjects (inconstantly in a third), the ability to produce separation in the presence of old disk degeneration and osteophyte formation has not been successful.[455, 456]

In summary, the coefficient of friction of a patient's body on a bed is such that any force less than 25 per cent of the body weight is incapable of producing traction on the lumbar spine, and even forces as high as 200 to 220 pounds for as much as 30 minutes cannot dependably produce intervertebral distraction.[455-457] The duration of pelvic traction as customarily employed ranges from continuous, if tolerated (usually with a traction force of 20 lbs. or less), to 20 minutes with cyclic or continuous traction on a split table using a force of 25 to 50 per cent of body weight.[143, 144] One can conclude that pelvic traction in a conventional hospital bed is an effective means of keeping a patient in bed and, provided it does not add to discomfort, may be of value for that purpose in the treatment of acute low back pain syndromes.[458] The question of the efficacy of friction-free pelvic traction methods (split-table) in reducing intradiscal or interfacetal derangements remains an open one and, like manipulative therapy, one that has strong advocates, many skeptics, considerable anecdotal support, and remains lacking in substantiation.

The use of *traction in cervical discogenic disease* or radiculopathy has had wider acceptance and more general use, although the status of its efficacy remains equally in doubt.[319] Cervical traction has been employed in a variety of positions and techniques. These include: supine with halter pulley and weights; supine with elevation of the head of the bed; seated with halter pulley and weights; supine, seated, with mechanically cycling traction; seated with relaxed, sagging upper body weight as the tractive force; with the distractive forces ranging from five to ten pounds (in the supine position) to as much as 300 pounds; and with duration of traction ranging from continuous, in the supine position, to cyclical traction for various periods, to a total traction session of as little as one minute in duration.[319, 330, 443, 447, 459-470] Most commonly a traction session lasts 20 minutes and is given once or twice daily, with the patient seated. The usual force or weight is 15 to 25 pounds.

It has been shown that measurable separation of the cervical vertebrae in healthy young males can be detected with a tractive force of 30 pounds after a duration of only seven seconds, but it has also been pointed out that in the presence of adhesions between nerve roots or the spinal cord and the dural canal, any vertebral separation may result in excessive tension on local structures.[470, 471] Out of this wealth of confusion of methodologies for cervical traction, each with its strong advocates but none with sufficient support for its efficacy, one has only highly empirical evidence as a basis for judgment as to whether or not to use cervical traction in any clinical setting.

Lacking sufficient scientific documentation for the efficacy of cervical traction in general, or any specific formula for the duration, amount, or optimal position for traction, this author can only pass along his personal bias in the selection of a simple, brief, and inexpensive cervical traction regimen.[153] For most patients with subacute to chronic neck pain secondary to trauma and discogenic disease, traction is readily applied with the patient seated with his or her side parallel to a door in a firm, armless chair. The traction device is suspended by a rope from an extension arm fitted over the top of a closed door. (See Fig. 31.) A halter is adjusted (commercial disposable halters are usually easily fitted) under the occiput and chin and attached to the suspended "spreader" bar with the patient sitting erect. The patient slides into a relaxed position with the neck in approximately 20 degrees of flexion. The tractive force then consists of a portion of the upper body weight (approximately 15 to 25 lbs.) and this is maintained for a period of five minutes once or twice daily.[472]

In general, traction is avoided in the presence of cervical inflammation (active rheumatoid arthritis), acute cervical trauma, and hemorrhage, or malignancy.[327, 445] Augmentation of cervical traction by concomitant cervical rotation has been recommended, but the risk of vascular occlusion has caused this exercise to be considered contraindicated.[48, 473-475]

During traction the patient should experience the pull of the halter equally under the mandible and the occiput, or slightly greater at the occiput, for maximum comfort, and traction should be discontinued if it increases discomfort. Stress on painful temporomandibular joints should be avoided and can be minimized by careful halter adjustment and positioning or by the use of a boxer's rubber mouth guard.[445-449, 451, 460]

Clearly there are a number of methods for applying cervical traction, and for any given patient one method may be preferred or better tolerated than another, but at the very least, the method described above provides most patients with an inexpensive "therapy" that can be continued at home without assistance after two or three brief supervised instruction sessions.

MASSAGE AND MANIPULATION

"During the T'ang Dynasty (A.D. 618–907) four kinds of medical practitioners were recognized: physicians, acupuncturists, masseurs, and exorcists."[476] As noted above, massage therapy has long been relegated to a place alongside of the physician, rather than integrated into his armamentarium. Nonetheless, massage through the ages and particularly in the Greco-Roman cultures has had a major place in therapeutics. Although a variety of massage techniques serving a fascinating variety of purposes have been developed, from the standpoint of rheumatology the primary purpose of massage is as an adjunct to obtaining muscle relaxation prior to stretching or strengthening exercises.

Massage as an effective means of inducing muscle relaxation of cramped or tight, tonically contracting muscles is widely accepted by the layman, but no studies of its efficacy in the management of musculoskeletal problems have been identified. The types and indications for the commonly used massage techniques include: stroking (effleurage), used superficially for its soothing effect and for deep muscle relaxation; compression (petrissage), as a kneading of tissues to stretch adhesions, mobilize edema, and also for muscle relaxation; and percussion (tapotement) as a stimulating counterirritant vibration or vigorous percussion. Massage is expensive in terms of therapists' time and effort. For practical reasons it is best restricted to those situations in which relaxation requisite for specific exercise cannot be obtained by simpler means such as the application of heat or cold, or by other muscle relaxation techniques.

The issue of *manipulation* is a more complex one and one that is fraught with considerably more prejudice. The potential and purported benefits of this relatively simple method of treatment challenges the utilization of the more conventional alternative measures that require a more prolonged or more hazardous therapy or periods of disability (e.g., the use of bed rest, medications, and surgery). To consider manipulation objectively one must separate this potential therapeutic approach from chiropractic teaching and practice. The rationale proffered by chiropractic dogma that the illnesses of man are caused by spinal subluxations and cured by spinal adjustments is unsubstantiated by scientific evidence.[477-479] Nonetheless, the diversion of as many as 200,000 patients per year through chiropractic or osteopathic manipulative therapies suggests the possibility that certain therapeutic alternatives may be unjustifiably ignored by the mainstream of medicine.[477-480]

Aside from the issue of whether or not manipulation, particularly as it is used for neck and back disorders, has therapeutic value, is the question of whether or not the risks preclude any serious consideration of this methodology. Manipulation of the cervical spine has been associated with documented cases of severe cerebrovascular and spinal cord damage, but the incidence of these complications would appear to be low, especially considering the large numbers of patients manipulated by nonphysician practitioners.[473, 481-484] Lumbar spinal manipulation, on the other hand, has apparently not been associated with any mortality and minimal morbidity, provided attention has been paid to obvious osseous defects.[473, 481-484]

Documentation of the efficacy of manipulation by rigorous scientific methodologies is insufficient, but serious consideration of the rationale for an approach to manipulative therapy has been given by a number of physicians, and there is now a society of physicians with a scientific interest in the science and technology of manipulation: the North American Academy of Manipulative Medicine.[458, 481, 485-490]

A detailed discussion of the rationale and methodology of manipulation is beyond the scope of this chapter. With regard to the cervical and lumbar spine, the methodological approach to manipulation involves positioning of the patient in the position of comfort to ensure relaxation so that muscles overlying a joint or a group of joints are placed at a maximum stretch, with the stretched muscles positioned so that they are mechanically disadvantaged (unable to forcefully resist the manipulative maneuver).[476, 490-492] With the patient thus positioned, a slight additional stretch — "thrust" — causes a distraction on the joint in question, often associated with an audible cracking sound.[476, 490-493] It is thought that the additional abrupt stretch on the already maximally extended muscle stimulates the Golgi tendon organs to induce further relaxation of the stretched muscle, thereby facilitating movement of the underlying articular structures.[490]

Pathological conditions amenable to manipulation are thought to be either displaced fragments of fibrocartilaginous disk material, facet joint synovium or capsule.[476, 490, 491, 494] These derangements are presumably restored to normal or premorbid relationships following manipulative distraction.[476, 491-492] It is also believed that the process of muscle stretching may relieve tonic ischemic phenomena considered to occur in muscles as a consequence of sustained protective muscle spasm.[476, 490-492] The applications of these techniques are limited to noninflammatory degenerative and discogenic disease. They are avoided in the presence of radiculopathy or underlying osseous defects such as severe demineralization, rheumatoid arthritis affecting the cervical spine, or primary or metastatic tumors.[327, 476, 490-492]

Similar manipulative techniques have been widely applied with less criticism, both with and without anesthesia, to peripheral joints. Manipulation is sometimes employed following immobilization after joint surgery or trauma; for mobilization of a chronic adhesive capsulitis of the shoulder; to a lesser extent for lateral epicondylitis ("tennis elbow"); and occasionally for MCP and PIP dysfunction associated with degenerative joint disease.[490, 494]

VAPO-COOLANT SPRAY AND LOCAL INJECTION THERAPY

The concept of a clinical entity characterized by foci of hyperirritable regions in muscle that when stimulated are capable of relaying pain to more distant regions (*trigger areas*) is poorly understood. It has been recognized for many years that the pain originating in deep myotomal structures has a distribution or body representation that differs from dermatomal patterns.[495-497] It has also been shown that predictable distribution patterns of pain can be elicited by local injections of as little as 0.5 to 1.0 ml. of 6 per cent saline into deep or myotomal tissue.[495-497] The "trigger areas" have been found to occur predictably in specified areas of muscles and these can be readily found by careful palpation.[498-502]

Painful muscle trigger areas are characterized by a palpable circumscribed area of muscle tenderness and induration, hence an apparent focal muscle contraction. It is of interest that the characteristic electromyographic activity noted with voluntary muscle contraction or with muscle spasms and cramps has not been consistently elicitable from these trigger areas.[498, 503-507] It is possible that loci of motor units within a muscle that are stimulated reflexly by remote pain protective phenomena are capable of maintaining a tonic muscle contraction with only a few motor units being activated at any one time. The tonic focal contraction sufficient to perpetuate the local tender area of muscle tension as well as refer pain is susceptible to treatment directed at the focus (or trigger area). When successful, persistent pain can be relieved, presumably by interrupting a pain cycle.[499-502, 508-510]

One of the methods that have had the greatest success in this regard is the *use of vapo-coolant sprays over the trigger area* and over the painful muscle.[498-502] Nonflammable fluori-methane is the vapo-coolant now preferred over flammable ethyl chloride.[499] The vapo-coolant spray technique for pain relief is an extension of the use of cold therapy as a counterirritant.[508] Vapo-coolant spray techniques can readily be taught for use at home. Vapo-coolant spray is administered with the jet approximately 33.0 cm. from the surface. A few seconds of spray over the trigger area and then tangential spraying consisting of one to three slow passes of the spray along the length of a muscle while it is in a stretched position are sufficient for one treatment.

Local anesthetic injections for focal muscle pain are a logical extension of their use in anesthesia. This method had wide acceptance as a useful therapeutic procedure for muscle "trigger" areas long before the use of local steroid injections.[502, 509, 510] There is, in fact, no evidence that steroids injected into these noninflamed trigger areas increase the effectiveness of the injection procedure.[485, 502, 509-512] Because there would appear to be no apparent advantage in the use of a steroid or potent anti-inflammatory agent locally in areas of reflex muscle irritability, one should not confuse this with the efficacy of steroid injections in myofascial, periarticular, and intra-articular disorders.

Local anesthetic spray or injections may be totally or partially effective or ineffective in relieving painful muscle trigger areas. A trial of two to three treatments for one to three weeks is justified if partial relief or increasing periods of temporary relief are obtained. The use of a vapo-coolant spray on the skin overlying any injection site is very helpful in reducing the discomfort associated with needle penetration.

TRANSCUTANEOUS NERVE STIMULATION (TNS)

It has long been recognized that various stimuli can alter pain perception. The specific effects of vibration stimulation as a counterirritation phenomenon have been demonstrated in both man and animals to raise the threshold to painful stimuli.[513] An outgrowth of this observation was the famous gate control system hypothesis for pain pathways which has served as a model for argument about the mechanisms of peripheral perceptions of pain.[514] More importantly for this discussion, the gate control theory provided a basis for the development of transcutaneous nerve stimulation techniques for pain relief.[514-517] Techniques as sophisticated as the use of dorsal spinal column stimulation for intractable pain and including percutaneous and transcutaneous nerve stimulation (TNS) have been designed to preferentially stimulate large diameter cutaneous afferent fibers in an effort to inhibit at the spinal cord transmission of painful stimuli.[516, 517] Thus far only one study utilizing a TNS technique has been rigorously designed to control placebo effects, and, although transient benefit was noted in neuropathies, no statistical benefit was observed at follow-up in any of the chronic pain syndromes studied.[119, 515-525]

Although TNS is moderately expensive, it is safe and easy to use, and has resulted in the reported relief of pain in many patients during its use. The ultimate role, if any, that transcutaneous nerve stimulation as a therapeutic modality should have is not yet established.[119, 515-524]

OPERANT CONDITIONING

The recurring issues of the lack of specificity of modalities used for relief of pain and the variety of approaches to relieve pain have recently led to two interesting approaches. Recognition that pain can be an all-encompassing psychophysiological phenomenon that is culturally conditioned has stimulated a proliferation of pain clinics and pain centers whose main theme seems to be the utilization of an operant conditioning methodology for managing chronic pain.[526-529] These highly structured, team-coordinated programs rely heavily on reconditioning the patient's attitude toward pain by rewarding the patient for "desirable" non-pain-focused behavior and either ignoring or "punishing" the patient for "undesirable" pain-oriented behavior.[527, 530, 531]

BIOFEEDBACK

Another aspect of pain that has been well recognized and can be related to psychosocial functioning is the effect of anxiety on muscle tension in chronic painful disorders.[116] The basic work of Basmajian on control over motor unit function has led to the use of electromyographic monitoring of muscle tension as a biofeedback phenomenon to assist patients in learning muscle relaxation as a method of obtaining pain relief.[405, 532-536]

It has been demonstrated that both healthy subjects and patients suffering from chronic neck and shoulder pain are unable to accurately perceive their level of muscle tension.[536] The inconsistency in achieving relief of pain and its associated muscle tension by the variety of therapeutic modalities previously described make it appealing to consider that the use of biofeedback may offer an additional rational and practical approach to relieve disorders in which chronic tonic muscle contraction appears to play an important pathogenetic role.[536] This again remains to be proved.

Another exciting potential new role has been reported for biofeedback in the control of the vasospasm of Raynaud's phenomenon.[537] If this is confirmed it will represent an important contribution of biofeedback to the management of a difficult therapeutic problem.

ACUPUNCTURE

Acupuncture thrust itself upon the Western scene in 1971 with considerable fanfare.[538] It offered a dramatic and potentially safe form of anesthesia for use in surgery, and a possible means of relief for a variety of disorders.[538, 539] In the field of rheumatology there are two early reports suggesting the value of acupuncture as a modality for pain relief in arthritis.[540, 541] Subsequent carefully controlled studies have not shown any specificity for acupuncture over placebo, and at this writing the hope that acupuncture may have tapped a new neurophysiological mechanism for relief of pain seems to be waning.[542-545]

ELECTRICAL STIMULATION

Eletrical current stimulation of motor nerves (faradic) or, in the case of denervation, of muscle itself (galvanic) has long been employed in therapeutic efforts. It has been suggested that muscle spasm attributable to painful joints may become relaxed after intermittent electrically induced contractions.[546] Pain reduction and relief of muscle spasm are reported but no controlled studies are cited.[546] In a controlled study in which electrical (faradic) stimulation sufficient to extend the knee against gravity was substituted for one of the quadriceps exercise sessions, no difference in the quadriceps strength was shown between those who received stimulation and those who did not.[546, 547]

A recent study utilizing electrical stimulation to overcome knee contractures in patients with upper motor neuron lesions demonstrated a change in the ratio of type I to type II fibers in the quadriceps, but this was not correlated with changes in strength.[546-548] It would appear that the use of faradic stimulation as an alternative massage technique may occasionally be justified.[546] Electrical stimulation of muscle contractions is widely employed as a therapeutic muscle training method in post-traumatic muscle injuries or tendon transplants.[546]

SELECTED READINGS BY TOPICS

(See also complete Bibliography on page 213.)

Heat, Cold, and Diathermy

376. Stillwell, G. K.: "Chapter 10. Therapeutic Heat and Cold," *in* F. H. Krusen, F. J. Kottke, P. M. Ellwood, eds., *Handbook of Physical Medicine and Rehabilitation.* 2nd Ed. Philadelphia: W. B. Saunders Co., 1971, Pp. 259–272.

413. Lehmann, J. F., Warren, C. G., Scham, S. M.: Therapeutic heat and cold. Clin. Orthop. Related Research, 99:207, Mar.–Apr. 1974.
419. Lehmann, J. F.: "Chapter 11. Diathermy," *in* S. Licht, ed., *Therapeutic Heat.* Baltimore: Waverly Press, Inc., 1958.

Hydrotherapy

440. Harris, R.: "Chapter 8. Therapeutic pools," *in* S. Licht, ed., *Medical Hydrology.* New Haven: E. Licht, 1963. P, 189.
441. Behrend, H. J.: "Chapter 12. Hydrotherapy," *in* S. Licht, ed., *Medical Hydrology.* New Haven: E. Licht, 1963. P. 239.

Traction

444. Farfan, H. F.: *Mechanical Disorders of the Low Back.* Philadelphia: Lea & Febiger, 1973. Pp. 220–221.
445. Harris, R.: "Chapter 12. Traction," *in* S. Licht, ed., *Massage, Manipulation and Traction.* New Haven: E. Licht, 1960. P. 223.
447. Judovich, B., Nobel, G. R.: Traction therapy, a study of resistance forces. Am. J. Surg., 93:108, Jan. 1957.
467. "Neckache and Backache." Proceedings of a workshop sponsored by the American Association of Neurological Surgeons in cooperation with the National Institutes of Health, Bethesda, Maryland. E. S. Guardjian, L. M. Thomas, eds. Springfield: Charles C Thomas, 1970.
472. Cailliet, R.: *Neck and Arm Pain.* Philadelphia: F. A. Davis Company, 1964. Pp. 79–82.

Manipulation

476. Licht, S.: *Massage, Manipulation and Traction.* New Haven: E. Licht, 1960. P. 104.
426. Ferris, B. G., Jr.: Environmental hazards. Electromagnetic radiation. N. Engl. J. Med., 275:1100, Nov. 1966.
491. Cyriax, J.: "Treatment by manipulation and massage," *in Textbook of Orthopaedic Medicine, Volume 1.* 6th Ed. Baltimore: Williams and Wilkins Co., 1975. Pp. 440–467, 699–719.

Vapo-coolant Spray

501. Travell, J.: Ethyl chloride spray for painful muscle spasm. Arch. Phys. Med., 33:291, May 1952.

Transcutaneous Nerve Stimulation

517. Pain Symposium. Congress of Neurological Surgeons. Surg. Neurol., 4:61, Jul. 1975.
525. Thorsteinsson, G., et al.: Transcutaneous electrical stimulation: a double-blind trial of its efficacy for pain. Arch. Phys. Med. Rehabil., 58:8, 1977.

Operant Conditioning

531. Fordyce, W. E. et al.: Operant conditioning in the treatment of chronic pain. Arch. Phys. Med. Rehabil., 54:399, Sept. 1973.

Chapter 8

PSYCHOSOCIAL, EDUCATIONAL, AND RECREATIONAL ASPECTS

PSYCHOSOCIAL FACTORS IN REHABILITATION

The dust is settling on the variety of psychological hypotheses relating to psychosomatic aspects of illness.[549-566] With regard to arthritic disorders, and in particular to rheumatoid arthritis, the consensus that is emerging is that the impact of pain and loss of function as a consequence of arthritic disorders will be manifested variously, depending on the patient's premorbid personality, his or her sex, and the psychosocial dislocation that occurs as a consequence of disease.[14, 94, 95-99, 566-575] The assessments stand in contrast to the organicity often associated with personality disorders in systemic lupus.[576] The problems relating to precision of methodologies, including the adequate definition of the case samples studied and the reproducibility of the psychological measuring instruments, have made interpretation of many of the psychological studies extremely hazardous.[18, 554, 561, 566, 577-581]

Patients with rheumatoid arthritis appear to *manifest certain common personality characteristics,* including depression, rigidity, and overconcern with bodily function, *but these have not been shown to be specific to rheumatoid arthritis* and would appear to be a consequence, not a cause of the disease.[562, 566, 571, 582] In an excellent editorial, Lipowski points out that in order to explain a person's psychological reaction to a disease, four classes of variables must be considered. These are: (1) the patient's personality and relevant aspects of his life history; (2) the patient's social and economic situation; (3) characteristics of the patient's nonhuman environment; (4) the nature and characteristics of the pathological process, injury, or physical disability, or all of these as they are *perceived and evaluated by the patient.*[583] He further stresses that the psychological response includes three dimensions: the intrapsychic (experiential), the behavioral, and the social (interpersonal).[583]

149

Severe crippling arthritis is a threatening disease. Pain, restriction of joint motion, and weakness lead to a poverty of movement and limitations of sensory and social experiences that can result in sensory deprivation stresses.[584-586] Crippling arthritic disorders can create actual or perceived personal loss and the depressive grieving reaction consequent to that loss, and it can open the possibility for secondary gains from the attentions that are engendered by illness and suffering.[14, 96-99, 570-575, 587]

A major link between the psychological status and the social functioning of the patient is his and his family's perception of what an appropriate sick role or response to pain should be. The psychological strength as well as physical, social, and economic resources that the patient can bring to bear will determine to what extent he will be successful in extricating himself from that role before he has closed his options to participate in the mainstream of society.[587-590]

In the past few years there has developed a wide recognition of the complexities of the interaction of pain and musculoskeletal disorders, particularly as they relate to back pain. The complexities of the psychological reactions to pain as well as the opportunities for therapy have opened up a new frontier in the comprehensive management of chronic musculoskeletal painful disorders.[590-604] Perhaps most innovative among the current approaches to the control of chronic and persistent painful disorders are the previously discussed operant conditioning, pain-behavioral-modification programs.[597, 605]

An important consequence of psychosocial dysfunction in arthritis and other disabling disease is *sexual dysfunction*. Loss of motion and pain on motion may create major problems in sexual relations, and this is most often recognized with hip joint involvement.[606] Sexual disability, however, can result from more subtle aspects of arthritic disorders, including depression, a feeling of being sexually undesirable because of obvious (and often subtle!) deformities, or even more indirectly because of misguided overprotection of the arthritic patient by the healthy sexual partner.[607-611] The clear documentation of the importance of sexuality and sexual function in the handicapped makes it imperative that the physician and allied health professional concerned with rehabilitation of the arthritic patients become conversant with their sexual problems. They must train themselves to be comfortable with discussions of sexual problems and with the alternatives and options that can be offered to the patient in order to enhance his or her opportunity to express sexuality.[79, 612, 613]

Another therapeutic innovation that has been rapidly expanding over the past two decades is *group therapy*. An outgrowth or collateral development is the proliferation of disease-oriented self-help groups for patients with categorical disease entities as well as for psychosocial dysfunction.[43, 559, 590, 614-623] A recent critical review of the *team care* and group methods in chronic disease management emphasized methodological problems involved in assessing their efficacy.[43] These include definition of objectives, process measures, outcome measures and accounting for variables such as the personalities of team members and group members, and the concurrent specific therapeutic and nontherapeutic inputs in the patient management process.[43] The overall impression is that group methods are of value, but they are probably too often functioning with nebulous objectives and goals in a loose and unstructured manner.[581] There is clearly a great need for additional research utilizing critical evaluative criteria on the group and team process.[43, 154, 581, 620, 623]

From the standpoint of rehabilitation, over and above the psychological considerations, there are a number of practical *social and economic needs* to be met by the arthritic patient. A partial list of these problems with some of the community resources that are available to resolve them has been compiled in the National Commission on Arthritis and Related Musculoskeletal Diseases report to the Congress of the United States, April, 1976.[8] An extremely comprehensive inventory of human needs has been developed which is inclusive enough to deal with, among other items: the adequacy of garbage disposals; criminal conviction record; air pollution; guide dogs for the blind; credit; deceptive, unlawful, unfair television, radio and stereo repair; infertility; smoking cessation programs; international travel; model plane flying; dunebuggying; and, under "Pets," rodents.[624, 625] Although the above inventory includes resources available in the Los Angeles area in which this survey was made, the problems surveyed and some of the resources identified are highly general and provide an excellent guideline that can appropriately be applied in a variety of settings.[624, 625]

An important attempt to quantify and score psychosocial function in a manner that is applicable to the problem-oriented medical record format and suitable for computerized data retrieval has been made.[74, 89, 626] Criteria have been established for communication capabilities, functional ability, support for family unit, ability to function in the home, educational and vocational potential, architectural barriers, and intellectual and emotional adaptability.[74]

EDUCATION IN REHABILITATION

In the broadest perspective the role of education in the rehabilitative process has several components. The juvenile arthritis patient's basic scholastic needs must be met in as normal a manner as possible so that he can grow to maturity with a minimum educational and psychosocial deficit. In the rehabilitative setting for both the adult and the child there is an additional need for education in specific functional skills and, in the case of the adult, for vocational retraining in order to provide marketable skills or professional expertise to the handicapped arthritic patient. The *arthritis patient education* component is somewhat more subtle, but in many ways more crucial if compliance with treatment and adjustment of life style are to be optimal and participation in quack cures is to be avoided.

The *"terminal educational objective"* of patient education is to modify the patient's (or family's) behavior in order to maximize the effectiveness of a therapeutic regimen.[627] It is usually not possible to achieve this objective by telling the patient what is wrong and what to do for treatment because of all the emotional factors and preconceptions that block communication and learning. Time for adjustment to new realities imposed by the arthritic disease or its treatment, time for repetition of content (preferably in various formats, e.g., discussions, books, audio-visuals) and reinforcement of desired behavior ("Good, your salicylate level is right on the money!"), and time for the patient's family or support groups to accept the patient's problems and participate constructively in their solutions must be spent wisely and well.

Each arthritis patient must come to an understanding of the nature of his disease, its implications, and all the requirements of his therapeutic regimen. This requires that the patient know the precise dosage schedules of all his medications, the possibilities of drug reactions, the precise exercise regimens, the nature of those steps necessary to protect his joints against abuse and further damage, and the use and maintenance of adaptive equipment and devices, as well as any therapeutic modalities that are prescribed so that he can properly take responsibility for his health maintenance.[628, 629] These aspects of education, which involve the physician, patient, family, and therapists, have too often been handled in a casual and unsophisticated manner. How often does the physician or therapist request feedback from the patient to determine if his thoughts were communicated and his technical jargon understood?

Modern educational psychology, learning theory, and methodology provide a wide range of resources to be used for the development of effective patient education programs.[627, 630-640] The fundamentals of education stress that at the time the patient is being "educated," consideration must be given to his psychological state, to family and social conditioning factors, and to acceptance or denial of disease as well as to the various techniques that can be utilized to present concepts and information.[641-643] In settings where a rehabilitation team is functioning, patient education goals and activities should be coordinated by team members.

There are a variety of patient education resources devoted to rheumatological disorders and their treatments that can be organized into individualized or group patient education curricula. These materials can be used in a private office, clinic, or ward and include audiovisual material, pamphlets and books, many of which can be obtained at no charge.[644, 645, 646] (See *Appendix B* for a sample patient education curriculum developed for occupational therapy.) Recently, much of the patient-oriented written material on arthritis and related disorders was screened for accuracy and organized into a library format designed to allow the patient to select reading materials relevant to his disease in order to inquire more effectively of his physician about problems related to his disorder and its regimens.[647]

Ultimately, the patient should know his diagnosis to avoid the anxiety-provoking speculation about what might be wrong (e.g., do I have a cancer or a contagious disease?), the precise treatment regimen including rest and recreational alternatives, the prognosis, and the therapeutic, psychosocial and economic resources available to maximize his ability to cope.[627] One cannot rely on patient education alone to guide patients into optimal therapeutic channels (witness the number of physicians who smoke), but without such patient education we cannot offer them protection against misguided therapies and quackery.

RECREATIONAL FACILITIES FOR THE HANDICAPPED ARTHRITIC

In considering recreation for patients who are disabled with arthritis, one must take into account the patient's interests, economic and social resources, energy level, mobility, tolerance to cold and drafts, predisposition to morning stiffness, and specific limitations imposed by joint inflammation, joint derangement, and susceptibility to further joint damage. For most patients with arthritic problems, swimming, with strokes modified to adapt to their disability or designed to increase their mobility and strength, is an ideal exercise. The combination of the warmth and particularly the buoyancy of the water facilitates joint movement and minimizes joint stress.

Diversional activities for the arthritis patient frequently include handcrafts. *Care must be given to ensuring that the craft activities for the patient with arthritis do not produce inordinate stress on involved joints.* Knitting and crocheting, particularly with small needles, may be a fine way to pass the time but a poor way to preserve finger joint integrity. Along with the encouragement of creative and constructive activities for the arthritis patient, attention should be given to proper positioning and, where needed, to the use of assistive devices to protect their joints.

Key factors in determining recreation choices for those patients who are on crutches, wheelchairs and other devices are access to public *transportation* and access to the recreation facility itself.[31] The "Dial-A-Cab" or local cars and minibuses operated by the American Red Cross, voluntary health organizations, and service clubs provide partial solutions to these problems for those patients who cannot utilize public transportation and do not have available private transportation.[238] *Travel by air* poses problems that include not only handling of baggage and boarding the plane, but layout barriers at air terminals and the individual airline policies with regard to assisting the handicapped as well.[648] For the handicapped person who must *travel in a wheelchair* there are a number of options for travel throughout the United States and abroad. Specific information is available regarding wayside stops, hotels and motels, restaurants and parks with facilities accessible to the wheelchair patient, theaters, museums, zoos, and other recreational facilities that have eliminated architectural barriers for the wheelchair patient or patients with significant ambulation problems.[238, 649]

The scope of recreational activities for patients with a variety of handicaps is limited only by the imagination and economic resources of the patient and therapist.[650] Recreational activities range from passive television viewing (which may require modification of the TV controls to permit independent usage) to a variety of games, bedside gardening, or outdoor gardening in raised soil beds accessible to wheelchairs and facilitated by adaptive garden tools.[237, 239, 651, 652] Conservation of energy and avoidance of joint stress must be a consideration in all activities, whether they be recreational or vocational, in which the patient with arthritis participates. In addition to psychological benefits, the potential for improved physical conditioning and function through recreational activities is great. It takes but little imagination to see the possibilities for the use of a loom as a means of exercising shoulders and elbows, a treadle-operated sewing machine for ankles, pitch-and-putt golf to increase walking tolerance, or sculpting in soft clay as a means of mobilizing stiff finger joints, but all such activities are best prescribed by a therapist skilled in the management of arthritic diseases.

SELECTED READINGS BY TOPICS

(See also complete Bibliography on page 213.)

Psychological Aspects

562. Wolff, B. B.: Current psycho-social concepts in rheumatoid arthritis. Bull. Rheum. Dis., *22*:656, Series 1971–1972.
566. Geist, H.: *The Psychological Aspects of Rheumatoid Arthritis.* Springfield, Ill.: Charles C Thomas, 1966. Pp. 11, 29.
569. Sternbach, R. A., Timmermans, G.: Personality changes associated with reduction of pain. Pain, *1*:177, 1975.
575. Freedman, A. M., Kaplan, H. I., Sadock, B. J.: *Comprehensive Textbook of Psychiatry, Vol. 2.* 2nd Ed. Baltimore: Williams & Wilkins, 1975. Pp. 1694–1704.
582. Meyerowitz, S.: "Chapter 7. The Continuing Investigation of Psychosocial Variables in Rheumatoid Arthritis," *in* A. G. S. Hill, ed., *Modern Trends in Rheumatology — 2.* London, 1971.
583. Lipowski, Z. J.: Psychosocial aspects of disease. Ann. Intern. Med., *71*:1197, Dec. 1969.

594. Szasz, T. R.: "The Psychology of Persistent Pain. A Portrait of L'Homme-Douloureaux," *in* A. J. Soulairac, et al., eds., *International Symposium on Pain.* New York: Academic Press, 1968. Pp. 93-113.

598. Grabias, S.: Topographical pain representations in the evaluation of low back pain. Resident paper presented at Rancho Los Amigos Hospital, Downey, Calif. March 29, 1974.

607. Ehrlich, G. E.: "Chapter 9. Sexual problems of the arthritic patient," *in* G. E. Ehrlich, Ed., *Total Management of the Arthritic Patient.* Philadelphia: J. B. Lippincott Co., 1973. P. 193.

608. Golden, J. S.: Sexuality and the chronically ill. The Pharos, *38*:76, 1975.

612. Greengross, W.: *Marriage, Sex and Arthritis.* London: The Arthritis & Rheumatism Council, S. G. Beaumont, Mill Lane, Harbeldown, Canterbury, Kent.

618. Sternbach, R. A.: *Pain Patients: Traits and Treatment.* New York: Academic Press, 1974. P. 105.

621. Rahe, R. H., O'Neil, T., Hagan, A., et al.: Brief group therapy following myocardial infarction: eighteen month follow-up of a controlled trial. Int. J. Psychiatry in Med., *6*:349, 1975.

Patient Education

627. Swezey, R. L., Swezey, A. M.: Educational theory as a basis for patient education. J. Chronic Dis., *29*:417, July 1976.

634. Gagné, R. M.: *The Conditions of Learning.* New York: Holt, Rinehart and Winston, 1970.

642. Davis, M. S.: Variations in patients' compliance with doctors' advice: An empirical analysis of patterns of communication. Amer. J. Public Health, *58*:274, Feb. 1968.

Recreation

648. Hogsett, S. G.: *Airline Transportation for the Handicapped and Disabled.* Chicago: National Easter Seal Society, 1972.

649. Annand, D. R.: *The Wheelchair Traveler.* Milford, New Hampshire: Douglas R. Annand, 1974.

Chapter 9 _____

CASE EXAMPLES OF REHABILITATION THERAPY

TABLE 9-1.   Rehabilitation Therapy Considerations

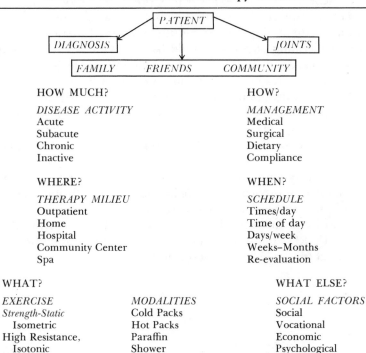

HOW MUCH?		HOW?
DISEASE ACTIVITY		*MANAGEMENT*
Acute		Medical
Subacute		Surgical
Chronic		Dietary
Inactive		Compliance

WHERE?		WHEN?
THERAPY MILIEU		*SCHEDULE*
Outpatient		Times/day
Home		Time of day
Hospital		Days/week
Community Center		Weeks–Months
Spa		Re-evaluation

WHAT?			WHAT ELSE?
EXERCISE	*MODALITIES*		*SOCIAL FACTORS*
Strength-Static	Cold Packs		Social
Isometric	Hot Packs		Vocational
High Resistance,	Paraffin		Economic
Isotonic	Shower		Psychological
Endurance	Tub		Educational
Low Resistance,	Whirlpool		Recreational
Repetitive	Pool		Transportation
Relaxation	Diathermy		
Stretch	Ultrasound		
Active ROM	TNS		
Active-Assisted	Biofeedback		
Passive	Electrical Stimulation		
	Massage		
	Traction		
	Vapo-coolant Spray		

WHY?	WHY NOT?
FUNCTION	*PRECAUTIONS*
ADL	Infection
Position	Tumor
Posture	Circulation
Casts	Pacemaker
Splints	Metal Implant
Assistive Devices	Sensation
Transfer/Gait	Weakness
Braces	Cardiopulmonary
Canes/Crutches	Status
Walkers	A.M. Stiffness
Wheelchairs	Drug Effects
Architectural Barriers	

REHABILITATION THERAPY

The schema (Table 9–1) which is presented prior to specific examples of therapy regimens for rheumatological disorders is designed to emphasize the multiplicity of considerations and therapeutic options that the prescribing physician should have in mind when outlining the program of management for the arthritis patient. Table 9–2 summarizes the usual referral resources for various aspects of the patient's management that need evaluation. The inclusive schema for arthritis rehabilitation therapy (Table 9–5), in addition to Tables 9–3 and 9–4, provides a format for specific rehabilitation therapy prescriptions, while Table 9–6 summarizes the precautions to be observed for the various therapy modalities.

A previously employed mnemonic device designed to outline the comprehensive approach to rehabilitation of the arthritic patient will again be used to help systematize the therapeutic approach for the sample cases that follow.[155] Two words are used as acronyms, the first being DISCORD (that which needs harmonizing), and the second, MEMORIES (therapies not to be forgotten).

Acronyms for Arthritis Assessment and Treatment

Assessment	*Treatment*
D–Diagnosis	**M**–Modality
I–Inflammation (on a 1 to 4 scale)	**E**–Exercise
S–Selection of joints	**M**–Movement or gait considerations
C–Chronicity	**O**–Occupational therapy
O–Other contributive medical problems	**R**–Rest
R–Restriction of joint mobility	**I**–Immobilization or splinting and bracing
D–Derangement of joints, such as dislocation or ankylosis	**E**–Education
	S–Social, psychological and vocational considerations

TABLE 9-2.   **Therapy Options**

	Evaluations
1. PHYSICAL THERAPY	(Modalities) Pain relief* (Exercise) Strength, endurance, joint mobility, posture (Mobility) Gait, transfer problems, transportation
2. OCCUPATIONAL THERAPY	(ADL) Activities of daily living, vocation, avocation, homemaking (Rest) Energy conservation, joint protection, body mechanics (Immobilization) Splints, assistive devices
3. EDUCATION	Knowledge of disease and treatment Learning capability, educational resources
4. SOCIAL	Economic status, options, and plans Family support, interpersonal relationships, sexual function Social and community resources
5. PSYCHOLOGICAL	Mental status, organic and functional alterations Drug dependence, suicidal tendency
6. VOCATIONAL	Employment status, alternatives and opportunities

*See Table 9-3.

TABLE 9-3.   **Selection Factors in Modalities for Pain Relief**

Pain Severity	Modality	Pain Localization	Comment
ACUTE	Ice pack Cold compress Ice massage	FOCAL	Avoid with cold intolerance or Raynaud's
	Warm moist compress		Most effective all around
	Hydrotherapy whirlpool tub tank pool		Warmth and buoyancy assist in stretching exercises
		GENERAL	
	Dry heat infrared bulb heating pad		Inexpensive for home use, portable, danger of short circuit
	Paraffin mud sand		Good palliative in PSS, RA*
	Diathermy microwave short wave ultrasound		Pacemaker and metal implant contraindicates**
CHRONIC		FOCAL	

*Paraffin only   **Short wave and microwave only

TABLE 9-4.   Guidelines for Therapy Prescriptions

1. Specify diagnosis. a. Indicate any special instructions or precautions for patient.

2. List the parts or area of body to be treated.

3. State *precisely the dosage* of each procedure to be used.
   a. Type of heat and length of application,
   b. The kind of massage and time to be spent in massage of each part,
   c. Type of exercise and purpose (muscle strengthening, muscle re-education, stretching, coordination, or relaxation).

4. Number and frequency of treatments during the day.

5. Direct what home measures are to be employed.
   a. Therapist to check patient's performance frequently.

6. Include date for re-evaluation by physician at which time he should:
   a. Ascertain that directions are carried out properly;
   b. Grade patient's performance;
   c. Add modifications, change frequency of treatments, etc.;
   d. Redetermine rest-exercise balance and coordinate total regimen;
   e. Furnish encouragement and provide support for patient's morale.

TABLE 9-5.   Inclusive Schema for Arthritis Rehabilitation Therapy

Patient Name_____, Age_____, Sex_____, Marital Status_____

Occupation_____, Employed_____, Health Insurance _____

Source of Referral_____, Education grade level_____

Inpatient_____, Outpatient_____

DIAGNOSIS: 1._____ 2._____ 3._____

Specific Problems (e.g., Cardiovascular): 1._____

2._____ 3._____

Functional (ADL) Evaluation _____

Splinting/Bracing – Location_____

＿＿＿＿＿＿＿ – Purpose_____

Assistive Devices – Equipment _____

＿＿＿＿＿＿＿ – Training_____

Energy Conservation and Joint Protection_____

Patient Education (Family Education)_____

Social Service Evaluation/Management_____

Psychological Evaluation/Management_____

Vocational Evaluation/Management_____

TABLE 9–5. Inclusive Schema for Arthritis Rehabilitation Therapy
(Continued)

THERAPY MODALITIES	____Massage	____TNS	
	____Cold	____Electrical Stimulation	
	____Microwave	____Ultrasound	____Hydrotherapy
	____Shortwave	____Hot packs	____Paraffin
	____Hubbard Tank, Pool	____Infrared	

CERVICAL/LUMBAR
      TRACTION: ____Intermittent
                       ____Constant   ____Body Suspension

                       pounds/kilos:_____time:_____

EXERCISE:	____Active	____Passive	____Active Assistive
	____Resistive	____Isometric	____Isotonic
	____Stretching	____Breathing Exercises	

GAIT TRAINING:	____No W.B.*	____Partial WB	____Full WB
	W.B.	____Right Leg	____Left Leg

AIDS:	____Crutches	____Walker	____Cane
	____Parallel Bars	____Brace(s)	____Prosthesis

EVALUATION: ____Muscle Strength Examination
                    ____Joint Evaluation
                    ____Functional Evaluation

PRECAUTIONS FOR THERAPY: Sensory, circulatory, metal implant, pacemaker, CNS disease, cardiorespiratory, acute inflammation, infection, tumor, osteoporosis, weakness, instability, psychological, drug effects

SCHEDULING OF THERAPY: MILIEU   Days/Wk.____, Total Wks. ____, Times/Day____,
Time of Day_____
Home, bed, gym, mat, pool, individual, group

SCHEDULING CONSIDERATIONS: Work/home/institution schedules, duration of a.m. stiffness, fatigue, pain, rate of improvement, motivation, transportation, cost.

PHYSICIAN'S SIGNATURE_____ DATE_____

*W.B. = weight bearing.
**See Precautions. Table 9–6.

TABLE 9-6. Precautions For Therapy Prescriptions

MODALITY	Impaired Sensation	Circulatory Deficiency	Metal Implant, or in Contact	Pacemaker	Cardiac, Respiratory, Cerebral Insufficiency	Acute Trauma, Inflammation	Infection	Tumor	Osteoporosis	Weakness, Endurance	Weight Bearing	Instability – Paralysis	Psychological Factors	Intellectual Factors	Economic Factors
LOCAL SUPERFICIAL* HEAT/COLD	R	R				R^h								R	
ULTRASOUND*	R	R	R			C	C	C							
DIATHERMY*	R	R	C	C		C	C	C							
HYDROTHERAPY WITH HEAT*	R	R			R	R		R						R	
GENERALIZED (TOTAL BODY) HEAT*	R	R			R			R		R		R		R	
TRACTION	R					R	R	C	R	R		R			
SPLINT/BRACE	R	R	R			R	R	R	R			R		R	
GAIT TRAINING	R				R	R	R			R	$R^{r/l}$	R	R	R	R
EXERCISE (PASSIVE, ACTIVE ROM/STRENGTH)		R	R		R	R	R		R	R		R			
MASSAGE/MANIPULATION					C^{cs}	C	C	C	R						R

C = Contraindications
R = Relative Contraindications or Special Considerations

h = heat
cs = cervical spine
r/l = right or left

*Specific operating instructions including dosage, exposure to moisture, duration of therapy, distance of energy source, or temperature of water must be adhered to rigorously.

CASE 1: Possible Psoriatic Arthritis, Subacute, Severe

A 24-year-old white woman with a history of morning stiffness, fatigue, occasional swelling of the left knee, and "bursitis" off and on in the right shoulder has for the past six weeks had severe generalized large and small joint inflammation. She has not been able to tolerate full doses of salicylates and thus far trials of two nonsteroidal anti-inflammatory drugs have provided only slight relief. The patient is married, has two young children, and works part time as a secretary to "help make ends meet." The current exacerbation occurred shortly after her father's untimely death in an auto accident.

Examination reveals the patient to be in significant distress from her generalized arthritis and she is obviously anxious and depressed. The positive findings are limited to the peripheral joints. There is slight erythema over the PIP and MCP joints of the hands. These joints, as well as the wrists, elbows, knees and ankles, are swollen and tender, and there is moderate restriction of their ranges of motion. Both shoulders are tender over the anterior capsules and are markedly restricted in motion, especially the right. The MTP joints of both feet are tender on palpation. Getting out of a chair and ambulation are performed with great pain and difficulty. There are no subcutaneous nodules, and no dermatitis is present, but psoriatic pitting of several finger nails is noted. The laboratory reveals only an elevated sedimentation rate (34 mm./hr. Wintrobe). Radiograms of all affected joints, the pelvis, and chest demonstrate soft tissue swelling, and some juxta-articular demineralization of the wrists and MCP and PIP joints is also noted.

Comment: This patient has a severe, persistent, generalized, symmetrical large and small joint inflammatory arthritis. Rheumatoid factor, ANA, and HLA-B27 tests are negative. Nail pitting suggests psoriasis, but there are no confirmatory findings (no DIP involvement, no typical or atypical rash, no periosteal proliferation). Psychological stress may have been a factor in precipitating this exacerbation, and social and economic concerns require immediate attention. Hospitalization for comprehensive care and control of this painful exacerbation should be arranged. (See acronym key page 158.)

Assessment:

D–Polyarthritis, possibly psoriatic, vs. RA
 I–Moderate–severe
S–Generalized in all peripheral joints
C–Subacute
O–Reactive depression
R–Moderate, all affected joints
D–None

Treatment:

M–Hubbard tank 30 minutes b.i.d. Hot packs to key painful joints for 20 minutes b.i.d. prn. Try paraffin to hands 20 minutes b.i.d. for pain relief.
 E–Active assisted range of motion performed gently b.i.d. to maintain mobility. These are best performed in midmorning and midafternoon after the Hubbard tank or hot packs. Two to three gentle stretches to achieve the maximum tolerated range in each joint are sufficient at each session.
M–Limited ambulation to lavatory assisted by platform crutches (with padded built-up hand grips). (See Fig. 66.) Fit for wheelchair as a basic short-term mobility aid. Teach transfers. Provide elevated toilet seat with grab bars.

O–Assess ADL. Provide assistive devices for grooming (long-handled comb), feeding (built up handles for silverware), hygiene (tooth paste dispenser), dressing (reacher, long-handled shoe horn, elastic shoe laces), bathing (shower seat, flexible hose attachments for shower head, bath soap holder). Teach joint protection and energy conservation techniques for dressing, grooming, etc. and begin instruction in these techniques for household activities. (See Figs. 67 to 71.)

R–At least 8 hours' bed rest at night and a one hour nap after mid-morning and afternoon exercise. Instruct in proper posture and positioning in bed and when seated. Prone position for 30 minutes twice daily to minimize hip flexion contractures. No pillows under the knees!

I–Provide positioning rest splints for fingers, wrists, knees, and ankles. A static "working" wrist-stabilizing splint should be provided for wear during activities. (See Fig. 52.) Posterior molded long leg splints extending from upper thigh to include entire foot with the ankle at 90 degrees should be worn as much as tolerated during rest to prevent knee and ankle contractures. Provide metatarsal pads in comfortable walking oxfords with crepe or soft ripple sole.

E–Explain nature of arthritic disease, and rationale for various therapies. Provide opportunities for patient and family to ask questions and clarify concepts. Emphasize need for compliance in all aspects of prescribed therapy. Anticipate use of possible quack remedies and warn of consequences.

S–Provide social services counseling to help arrange for child care and homemaking assistance during and following hospitalization. Assess health insurance and possible supplemental support for medical and household expenses. Provide family counseling to minimize impact of disability on all concerned. Contact community agencies and arthritis support groups to explore additional emotional and financial resources. Request psychiatric consultation re depression and need for formal psychotherapy or pharmacological therapy. Counsel patient and spouse on sexual problems and concerns. Explore possible vocational alternatives if present job (demanding almost constant typing) cannot be resumed.

CASE 2: Rheumatoid Arthritis, Chronic, Multiple Small Joints

A 33-year-old housewife with classic rheumatoid arthritis of seven years' duration has slowly progressive joint disease affecting the PIP and MCP joints of both hands, both wrists and the MTP joints bilaterally. The inflammatory component of her disease has been under control since she was started on gold medication 1½ years previously, but her fingers are stiff and difficult to use in the morning. She has difficulty with hand function because of finger deformities, and experiences pain on ambulation due to callosities under the balls of her feet and over the dorsi of her toes.

On examination the patient appears mildly chronically ill but in no acute distress. She has obvious swan neck deformities of the index and middle fingers on both hands, a boutonnière deformity of the right fifth finger, and instability of the PIP joint of the right thumb. Ulnar deviation of the fingers is mild and there is moderate restriction of wrist motion bilaterally. The metatarsal heads are subluxated on the plantar surfaces and there are dense callosities underlying them. All the toes manifest cock-up deformities and there are callosities overlying the PIP joints of the second and third toes of both feet. The laboratory reveals a rheumatoid factor of 1:1250; a Wintrobe sedimentation rate of 25 mm. per hour; a hemoglobin of 12 gm. per 100 ml. Radiograms confirm the above-described deformities and also show mild erosive changes and narrowing in the same joints.

Comment: This patient's arthritis is under good control although she still has discomfort and functional disability as a consequence of the previous joint damage. The fixed deformities preclude correction with conservative measures and the need is to improve her ability to function and relieve discomfort pending arrangements for MTP arthroplasties and subsequent hand surgery. (See Acronym key page 158.)

Assessment:

D–Rheumatoid arthritis

 I–±

S–PIP, MCP, wrists, IP joint, right thumb, and MTP joints, bilaterally

C–Chronic

O–Noncontributory

R–Moderate in all affected areas

D–Boutonnière deformity, right fifth finger; subluxation and instability, IP joint, right thumb; swan neck deformity, index and middle fingers, both hands; mild volar deformity, left wrist; MTP subluxation and cock-up toe deformities, both feet; erosive joint disease in all the above areas.

Treatment:

M–Hot soaks or paraffin to hands for 10 minutes in A.M. to relieve stiffness

 E–Active range of motion to all affected upper extremity joint areas b.i.d.

M–Prescribe orthopedic shoes with high wide toe box and metatarsal pads to relieve MTP plantar stress and PIP pressure dorsally.

O–Assess household activities and other activities of daily living. Teach joint protection to minimize stress on fingers and wrists. Provide elastic shoe laces.

R–Eight hours' sleep at night and 30 to 60 minute nap daily.

I–Static working wrist splint for right hand during stressful activities. Splint PIP joint, right thumb, to stabilize during functional activity. (See Figs. 52 and 54.)

E–Teach patient the value of joint protection. Explain the benefits and risks of proposed surgery. Review medication regimen.

S–Plan for assistance with heavy household chores. Discuss with patient and spouse issues relating to physical appearance, joint deformities, and sexuality.

Comment: This woman has chronic destructive and deforming rheumatoid arthritis, which is near remission on gold therapy. Her chief problems are related to residual deformities, but she needs instruction in further protection and optimum usage of the joints that have sustained damage in order to prevent further deformity and exacerbation of her smoldering disease. Surgical treatment will probably relieve her foot problem and may improve function as well as cosmesis in the hand. Nonetheless, stresses to the small joints and wrists should be kept minimal, hence the need for instruction in joint protection and recommendation for the elastic shoe laces to minimize finger stress when tying the shoes. Ulnar deviation is not progressing or painful, nor is it posing a functional or cosmetic problem. Joint protection techniques are sufficient and no corrective splint is prescribed. (See Fig. 53.) Consideration to the patient's total life style is essential because of the chronicity of her problems.

CASE 3: Reiter's Syndrome, Subacute, Painful Weight-Bearing Joints

This patient is a 24-year-old man with a history of moderate to severe painful swelling of both ankles, the right heel, and both knees, beginning two months previously. At the onset there were an associated mild conjunctivitis and a nonspecific urethritis, which subsided without treatment after two weeks. Because of pain in the left knee, right heel, and ankle, the patient could ambulate for only short distances with great difficulty.

Examination was essentially normal except for a subsiding balanitis and the articular involvement. There was two plus swelling, heat, and tenderness in the left knee, which lacked 20 degrees of extension and 30 degrees of flexion. There was moderate atrophy of the left quadriceps muscle. The right ankle was moderately swollen, slightly warm, and moderately tender, and lacked 15 degrees of flexion and extension. The anterior surface of the calcaneus at the insertion of the plantar fascia was markedly tender on deep palpation. Laboratory revealed a Wintrobe sedimentation rate of 25 mm. per hour and a positive HLA-B27 antigen. Radiograms showed soft tissue swelling of the left knee and right ankle and irregular periosteal proliferation on the anterior surface of the right calcaneus.

Comment: Persistent involvement of the left knee and right heel and ankle in this patient with Reiter's syndrome precludes useful ambulation.

Assessment:

D–Reiter's syndrome

 I–2+

S–Left knee, right ankle, right heel

C–Subacute

O–None

R–Moderate, left knee and right ankle

D–Potential calcaneal spur on right

Treatment:

M–Whirlpool or tub to both lower extremities, 20 minutes, at 30 to 40 degrees C., b.i.d.

E–Active-assisted, ranging to left knee and right ankle, b.i.d. General conditioning activities (swimming).

M–Teach alternating four-point crutch gait for short distance ambulation; prescribe wheelchair for prolonged travel.

O–Arrange dressing, grooming, and other activities to minimize weight bearing during standing or ambulation.

R–Ad lib.

I–Posterior molded splint extending from upper thigh to and including left foot, with left ankle at 90 degrees to maintain maximum knee extension at night and when resting during the day. Below-knee weight-bearing brace with SACH heel, rocker sole, and horseshoe heel insert on right shoe. (See Figs. 58 and 59.)

E–Explain nature of Reiter's disease and prognosis.

S–Discuss possible change of vocation to avoid prolonged standing if lower extremity involvement proves to be slow in responding.

Comment: Reiter's syndrome is generally self-limiting, but persistent lower extremity involvement can cause considerable disability due to impaired ambulation. The below-knee weight-bearing brace can be extremely useful in patients with severe ankle and hind foot involvement to minimize weight-bearing stress and facilitate ambulation. The posterior molded leg splints should be adjusted weekly as the knee flexion contracture is being overcome.

CASE 4: Ankylosing Spondylitis, Mild

A 24-year-old white male has had increasing back pain for the past four months. The onset of back pain two years previously was associated with alternating pains in the buttocks. This has persisted, with periods of varying degrees of severity, until the most recent and persistent episode. He had an unexplained swelling in the left knee for a period of three weeks two years ago but no other complaints.

Examination reveals a fairly well-developed young man in mild distress. Restriction of lumbar motion is almost complete. Chest expansion is 1½ inches. There are no other joint abnormalities and no visual abnormalities, and no murmurs are heard. The laboratory reveals a Wintrobe sedimentation rate of 23 mm. per hour. Rheumatoid factor is negative. B27 antigen is present. Radiograms demonstrate bilateral sacroiliitis and squaring of the anterior margins of the second and third lumbar vertebrae with early syndesmophyte formation.

Assessment:

D–Ankylosing spondylitis

 I–2+

S–Sacroiliac, lumbar and costovertebral

C–Chronic

O–Transient knee involvement without sequelae

R–Loss of lumbar motion and chest expansion

D–Fusion of sacroiliac joints and early fusion of lumbar vertebrae

Treatment:

M–Hot tub or shower prior to exercise

 E–Chest expansion, back extension and stretching and back extensor strengthening exercises (See Figs. 18, 19, 22, and 34.)

M–No problems

O–Arrange activities to avoid low back stress. Teach patient postural cues. Provide firm mattress with board and no pillow. Encourage stretching during self-care activities, such as dressing. Teach patient to measure height each month to detect any forward bowing of the spine and to measure distance between the fingertips and the floor on attempted spinal flexion once each month.

 R–See above. Prone positioning is not essential with normal hip mobility.

 I–None

 E–Explain nature of ankylosing spondylitis and the need to avoid stress to back, and for periodic ophthalmological, rheumatological-medical follow-up. The basis for the nonsteroidal anti-inflammatory drug regimen and the implications of the B27 associated genetic trait must be taught.

 S–Advise re adopting a lifestyle to avoid periods of excessive physical stress and permit maximum mobility and position change at work.

Comment: The patient was placed on nonsteroidal anti-inflammatory medication for control of symptoms. His disease has been limited thus far to spinal involvement with associated restriction of chest expansion. Thus far he has had a fairly mild course of ankylosing spondylitis, the discomfort from which should be well controlled by nonsteroidal anti-inflammatory medication. With proper emphasis on posture and exercise he should avoid significant deformity. Periodic follow-up examinations are necessary to detect any progression, peripheral joint involvement, or ophthalmological or cardiac complications which would require additional therapeutic measures. The profound morning stiffness may be relieved by having the patient assume a crawl (on hands and knees) position in bed and from that posture to first rock back and forth, then reach forward with his arms, sit back on his heels, and reach backward with his legs alternately, or to actually crawl as a general loosening up regimen. (See Figs. 32 and 33.)

CASE 5: Severe Ankylosing Spondylitis with Hip, Knee and Shoulder Involvement

A 29-year-old male machinist has had progressive stiffening of his entire spine for five years. Pain has been considerably improved by indomethacin 25 mg. t.i.d., but hip mobility has become markedly compromised. Shoulder mobility has been gradually decreasing on the right, and moderately painful, remitting knee effusions have become more persistent. He has had multiple episodes of iritis, but these have thus far been well controlled with local steroid eye drops.

Examination reveals a thin chronically ill–appearing young man with obvious marked restriction of spine mobility, who stands throughout his interview and most of the examination because of his inability to sit in the available chairs. His vital signs are normal. A slight irregularity of the right pupil is noted, but there is no gross impairment of vision. Temporomandibular motion is intact and painless. The neck motion is limited to 20 degrees of right or left rotation and there is a similar restriction of flexion and extension. There is a 5 cm. gap between the occiput and the wall when standing (with his spine flat against the wall). Chest expansion is 2 cm. Schober's test reveals no lumbar motion in flexion-extension, and there is also no lumbar or dorsal rotation. The dorso-lumbar spine is straight, but there is a 30 degree flexion contracture of both hips, causing him to stand with his knees in partial flexion in order to look straight ahead. Both knees are mildly swollen, warm and tender, but there is full active and passive knee mobility. The musculature is generally underdeveloped, but there is no weakness on manual muscle testing, nor is any neurological deficit noted.

Range of motion of the right hip in flexion-extension is 70–30 degrees and in internal-external rotation 0–20 degrees, with abduction restricted to 10 degrees. There is moderate pain on all movements of the right hip. The left hip has similar flexion-extension, and approximately twice the mobility of the right in all other planes. The right shoulder can actively abduct and flex 90 degrees, and passively 110 degrees, and internal and external rotation are 30 degrees and painful at the extremes of movement. The shoulder musculature on the right is atrophic when compared to the left. The significant laboratory findings are a Wintrobe sedimentation rate of 34 mm./hour, and a positive HLA-B27.

Radiograms reveal a "bamboo" spine with ankylosis from C_2 to S_1, essentially obliterated sacroiliac joints, erosion and marked narrowing of both hips, and effusions of both knees. There is slight narrowing of the right glenohumeral joint. Osteoporosis is generalized.

Assessment:

D–Ankylosing spondylitis

 I–Mild to moderate

S–Entire spine, right shoulder, both hips, both knees

C–Chronic

O–Iritis

R–Both hips, right shoulder, spine below C_2

D–Ankylosed spine, and sacroiliac joints, marked destruction of both hips

Treatment:

M–Warm pool for range of motion exercises. Hot shower before limbering up.

 E–Gentle range of motion exercises for hips to preserve motion b.i.d. Codman exercises b.i.d. for right shoulder, followed by gentle active-assisted stretching exercise with reciprocal pulley or stick for right shoulder. (See Figs. 12 to 16.) Isometric strengthening of shoulder abductors (deltoid) 6 seconds b.i.d. in position of comfort and of internal and external rotators. (See Fig. 46.) Range of motion, both hips, in pool, and walking and swimming in pool daily to maintain mobility and increase strength of hip musculature. Use side stroke (right side up) to protect right shoulder. Six seconds of quadriceps isometrics b.i.d. (See Fig. 49.) Deep breathing exercises at this stage are rarely able to increase intercostal excursion but sometimes appear to reduce chest pain. *Note:* A local steroid injection might expedite restoration of shoulder mobility.

M–Provide forearm crutches to relieve stress on hips and knees, but watch for increased stress on right shoulder. Remove all throw rugs or potential hazards that might trip patient. Advise auto with wideview rear-vision mirror, and semireclining car seat. If necessary, a van with customized seating and a large door to facilitate entry is recommended. Provide semireclining wheelchair for mobility where walking or driving is not feasible.

O–Provide bar stool type seats or specially modified saddle seating on a stool for household and work. Raise all counters, provide grab bars in showers, near toilet and to assist in transfer from bed. Provide a raised toilet seat. Teach energy conservation and joint protection. Organize household and work activities to minimize stress and to maximize accessibility.

Recommend wearing loafers, or shoes with elastic laces. Provide reachers with hooks and pincers to assist in dressing and retrieving dropped objects. (See Fig. 71.) Provide prism glasses to facilitate reading in bed.

R–Prone position on firm mattress 30 minutes b.i.d. to minimize progression of hip contractures. Use minimal pillow, sufficient to support the occiput when supine and to provide some lateral neck support when folded for side-lying.

I–None

E–Explain ankylosing spondylitis and the status of his disease. Reinforce need for ophthalmological follow-up and general medical (cardiac) as well as musculoskeletal evaluations. Discuss implications of the genetic marker HLA-B27. Reinforce importance of exercise regimen.

S–Assist patient and employer in finding light work in his trade. A proper stool will permit him to work in a seated position and minimize stress on his knees. Vocational retraining may be required to develop special skills in light work machine trades. Give patient the opportunity to verbalize on his frustrations. Discuss sexual problems with candor and be prepared to offer specific recommendations – e.g., the reverse "missionary" position to minimize shoulder stress.

Comment: This young man has severe and advanced ankylosing spondylitis. His spine is fixed in good position, although he has a forward-thrusting neck. His hips are severely involved and the hip flexion contractures are causing additional stress to his knees. The marked restriction of both spine and hip motion makes sitting in ordinary chairs or on a toilet almost impossible. Driving a car is extremely difficult and actually dangerous without adequate modifications. The hips will require surgery for useful function; the right shoulder has moderate restriction of both active and passive motion, but there are only minimal radiographic changes and local therapy may restore useful function.

CASE 6: Septic Arthritis, Acute, Elbow

A 23-year-old female patient under intensive steroid and immunosuppressive therapy for systemic lupus erythematosus developed severe pain, heat, and swelling in the left elbow. Aspiration produced purulent material which on culture revealed *Staphylococcus aureus.*

Assessment:

D–Staphylococcal sepsis

I–4+

S–Right elbow

C–Acute

O–Systemic lupus erythematosus, steroid and immunosuppressive therapy

R–Joint immobile because of pain

D–None

Treatment:

M–Cold compresses p.r.n.

E–Gentle assisted range of motion in flexion, extension, pronation, and supination once daily following cold compress

M–Does not apply

O–Arrange bedside personal effects to accommodate affected right arm and I.V. in left arm

R–Ad lib

I–Posterior molded splint to upper one-third of right arm extending to wrist, with elbow positioned at 90 degrees of flexion and mid-range of pronation/supination

E–Provide general information about SLE and specific knowledge about present episode. Reinforce drug regimen details, including side effects.

S–Discuss prognosis with family and orient family to provide emotional support during this acute complication as well as the chronic phase of SLE.

Comment: Prompt antibiotic therapy with daily aspiration of purulent material, even in immunosuppressive drug–treated patients, should result in a cure of the septic process. Immobilize until abatement of pain permits gentle active-assisted ROM exercises once daily. As inflammation subsides, range of motion exercises can be increased to two to three times daily. (See Figs. 10 and 11.) Warm compresses may be more helpful in pain relief in the later phase of healing. As long as flexion is maintained by range of motion exercise, casting or posterior molded splinting can be gradually modified to assist in restoration of elbow extension. When inflammatory signs and symptoms are minimal, exercise to restore mobility can be done at increasingly more frequent intervals, up to hourly if the exercise is not associated with increased pain and swelling. Isometric exercises 6 seconds b.i.d. to biceps, triceps, pronators, and supinators are added after ROM regimen is established. (See Figs. 43 to 45.) When full mobility has been restored, ROM exercise therapy can be discontinued, but home strengthening regimen should be continued for 12 weeks.

CASE 7: Acute Arthritis, Pseudogout, Left Ankle

A 47-year-old man noted swelling in the left ankle for two days, with increasing pain during the past 24 hours. He had had a previous similar episode involving the left knee, and a diagnosis of idiopathic chondrocalcinosis and pseudogout was made. Pain in the left foot was so severe that he could not tolerate weight bearing. Aspiration of the ankle produced typical calcium pyrophosphate crystals but the laboratory revealed no additional abnormalities. Radiograms of the ankle were negative. Previous x-rays of both knees had shown calcification in the menisci.

Assessment:

D–Pseudogout

  I–4+

S–Left ankle

C–Acute

O–No evidence of diabetes, hyperparathyroidism, hemachromatosis or Wilson's disease.

R–Maximal

D–None

Treatment:

M–Trial of cold compresses for pain relief

  E–None

M–Teach non-weight-bearing (left leg), 3-point-crutch gait

O–None

R–Ad lib

  I–A padded posterior molded splint or foot board may provide additional comfort.

  E–Patient has already been instructed in the nature of his disease and the need for the anti-inflammatory medication he is receiving, as well as side effects of the medication.

S–Does not apply

Comment: Pseudogout is usually acute and self-limiting in nature. It is generally aggravated by local heat applications. The acute episodes per se rarely lead to residual joint damage or deformity. With the subsidence of pain, the patient can return to normal weight bearing and will not require a specific exercise regimen. Chronic chondrocalcinosis, in contrast to the acute episodes, can be associated with a progressive destructive degenerative joint disease.

CASE 8: Scleroderma (Progressive Systemic Sclerosis, Mild)

A 42-year-old housewife has noted increasing tightness of the skin on her hands and forearms for two to three years. She has noted cyanosis of her fingers intermittently, particularly on exposure to cold, for about five years. She has suffered moderate joint pain in her hands, with occasional joint swelling, for one year. During the past year she has also noted occasional dysphagia. She has a 20-year history of cigarette smoking (one pack per day).

On examination the vital signs are normal, slight tightness of the perioral skin is noted, and marked tethering of the skin from the distal forearm to the finger tips is observed. There is slight atrophy of the fingertip pads, and a few pitted 1 mm. scars on the finger tips are seen. There is a 15 degree flexion contracture of all the PIP and DIP joints. The MCP, PIP, and DIP joints flex to 70 degrees. There is tenderness on firm palpation of the PIP joints on both hands and over the right index MCP joint. No other abnormalities are noted except for a transient cyanosis of the right fourth and fifth fingers. The Wintrobe sedimentation rate is 25 mm./hr., and all other laboratory examinations are normal. Radiograms of the hands reveal soft tissue atrophy and slight general bony demineralization. Hypomotility was noted on the esophagram.

Assessment:

D–Progressive systemic sclerosis

 I–Mild MCP and PIP

 S–Hands MCP and PIP

C–Chronic

O–Raynaud's, dysphagia

R–MCP and PIP, skin of hands and face

D–None

Treatment:

M–A trial of paraffin for 20 minutes once or twice daily may give relief of joint discomfort, create an apparent softening of the skin and facilitate ROM exercise.

E–Active-assisted for finger joints. Range each joint three to five times at least b.i.d. (See Figs. 2 to 6.)

M–Not relevant

O–Teach joint and skin protection. Avoid hand exposure to cold atmosphere and objects. Build up handles to facilitate grasp. Provide cotton gloves for hand protection when exposed to cold.

R–Caution regarding general overfatigue or excessive stress to joints.

 I–Trial of spring wire Bunnell "knucklebender" splints, 20 minutes t.i.d. on MCP and PIP joints. (See Figs. 7 and 8.) If tolerated, continue for at least two weeks. If ROM of treated joints is improving, continue until maximum motion is achieved.

E–Advise to quit smoking. Reinforce hand protection. Discuss nature of disease and prognosis with patient and family.

S–Explore tension-causing conflicts at home. Provide ongoing emotional support.

Comment: The patient has an insidiously progressive systemic sclerosis with contractures in her finger joints and Raynaud's phenomenon associated with early atrophic finger tip scarring. Avoidance of cold-induced ischemic damage to the hands, and maintenance of hand function are the crucial objectives of therapy.

CASE 9: Cervical Discogenic Disease with Strain

A 56-year-old male postal worker recently developed increasing pain and stiffness in his neck, particularly aggravated by attempts to rotate the neck to the right. He has had similar but less severe complaints on several occasions in the past 10 years. He has been aware of eye strain but has not yet gotten around to having his eyes examined. Examination reveals tenderness in the right paracervical musculature with moderate restriction of cervical rotation and lateral flexion bilaterally, more marked on the right. There is no neurological deficit. X rays show mild discogenic disease between C_5 and C_6 and C_6 and C_7.

Assessment:

D–Cervical discogenic disease

 I–None

S–C_5, C_6, and C_7

C–Subacute to chronic

O–Eye refraction problems, sitting posture

R–Moderate on cervical lateral flexion and rotation bilaterally, greater on right.

D–None

Treatment:

M–Hot compress followed by cervical traction, 5 minutes, seated with body suspension, b.i.d. (See Fig. 31.)

E–Defer (cervical mobilization and isometric exercises of neck flexors and extensors) until pain has further subsided. (See Figs. 30 and 47.)

M–Not relevant

O–Evaluate to adjust desk height and lighting for work, and posture during activities of daily living (watching TV, driving).

R–Instruct in relaxation techniques; use small pillow or dumbbell-shaped pillow (permits lateral support on side-lying) at night.

 I–Defer the use of cervical collar for one week unless symptoms intensify.

E–Advise re posture and work habits to avoid neck stress, particularly emphasizing the need to interrupt sustained activities before significant pain develops.

S–Explore tension-provoking conflicts at work and at home.

Comment: The patient's occupation requires prolonged desk work and intensive reading. Both stressful neck position and eye strain may be contributing factors.

CASE 10: Cervical Discogenic Disease, with Acute C_6 Root Compression

A 43-year-old housewife noted discomfort in her right shoulder and arm while stacking books on a high attic shelf. The following day the arm pain was more severe, and there was moderate to severe neck pain and stiffness. Examination reveals moderate restriction of neck motion in all planes and marked restriction of cervical extension, right lateral flexion and rotation. These movements precipitate severe neck and shoulder pain. There is diffuse tenderness of the posterior neck musculature and local accentuation of tenderness with percussion on the spine of C_6, and on deep palpation of the low cervical paraspinous muscles and the suprascapular musculature just superior to the superior-medial angle of the right scapula. Full abduction and rotation of the shoulder are restricted by pain. The shoulder rotator muscles and the biceps on the right are perceptibly weaker than on the left (grade $5-$). The right biceps and brachioradialis reflexes are slightly hypoactive. There is patchy hypesthesia and hypalgesia over the lateral aspect of the distal half of the forearm. Radiograms of the cervical spine reveal only a slight reversal of the normal cervical lordotic curve. No EMG was done because of the short duration of symptoms.

Assessment:

D–Acute C_6 radiculopathy, right side, secondary to cervical disk protrusion

I–Minimal, associated with acute intrinsic trauma

S–Right C_6 root, C_5–C_6 disk and cervical paraspinous muscles, as well as right suprascapular muscle "trigger area" and right shoulder, arm and forearm

C–Acute

O–None

R–Moderate to severe on motion of the neck. Early restriction of right shoulder motion due to pain.

D–Weakness of shoulder musculature and biceps

Treatment:

M–Cold or warm compresses can be tried p.r.n. for relief of pain, but only if careful maintenance of neutral or least painful cervical position is observed by supine or side-lying positioning with firm head support or traction. Intermittent seated traction, 15 to 20 lbs. or body suspension for 5 to 20 minutes with neck in mild flexion and in position of maximum comfort, should be tried for pain relief. (See Fig. 31.) Supine traction, sustained, or as tolerated, for pain relief with weights of 5 to 7 lbs. should be instituted if pain or neurological signs and symptoms increase.

E–Gentle active-assisted range of motion twice daily to maintain shoulder motion and if possible restore lost motion. Ice packs to neck and shoulder prior to exercise may inhibit painful muscle spasm.

M–Restrict ambulation to minimal household activities, e.g., to bathroom or dining room.

O–Defer until pain and neurological status stabilize. (See *Case 9, Cervical Discogenic Disease with Strain.*)

R–Use dumbell-shaped pillow with firm lateral head support for side lying and minimal occipital support for supine position. Avoid prone position. Wear Philadelphia collar in bed until cervical pain and neurological signs and symptoms have been stable for at least two weeks. (See Fig. 61; see Tables 5–1 and 5–2.)

I–Fit with SOMI or similar brace for daytime activities and Philadelphia collar for use in bed. (See Fig. 62.) When pain and neurological signs and symptoms have stabilized, use Philadelphia collar alone if patient prefers. With refractory or progressive symptoms, hospitalization and continuous traction should be instituted, with close coordination by a neurosurgical consultant.

E–Explain nature of problem and rationale for immobilization. Point out that prognosis is ultimately favorable in most cases.

S–The impact of restricted activities on personal and vocational activities should be discussed and assistance in planning for short- and long-term socioeconomic adjustments initiated.

Comment: This patient has developed an acute C_6 root lesion, apparently precipitated by disk stresses from sustained cervical hyperextension. Stabilization of the cervical spine and the neurological deficit is the major concern, and pain relief is essential.

CASE 11: Lumbosacral Strain, Acute, Subsiding

A 43-year-old housewife bent over to pick up a box of laundry soap from under the sink and experienced a severe, diffuse low back pain. She has been at bed rest for the past week and has no discomfort at rest at this time, but she has moderate distress on getting in and out of bed. She can sit or stand for only about 20 minutes without experiencing a mild to moderate recurrence of low back pain and stiffness. Examination reveals moderate restriction in all planes of lumbar spine movement, and straight leg raising produces pain in both posterior thigh areas at 80 degrees of hip flexion. The neurological examination is within normal limits. There is a 3/4 inch shortening of the right leg. Radiograms reveal no abnormalities.

Assessment:

D–Lumbosacral strain

I–±

S–Lumbosacral juncture

C–Acute, subsiding

O–Tight hamstring muscles, general deconditioning, short right leg

R–Consistent with lumbar muscle spasm

D–None

Treatment:

M–Hot packs, 20 minutes, every two hours

E–Begin pelvic tilts and knee chest exercise; after 48 hours, if tolerated, commence abdominal isometric exercises. (See Figs. 23, 35 to 37.)

M–Provide 1/2 inch heel lift on right. (See Fig. 60.)

O–Provide elevated toilet seat and a firm armchair. Teach body mechanics to avoid stress on lumbar spine in transferring in and out of bed, in and out of chair, and during dressing. (See Figs. 40 to 42.) Provide a firm car seat support and teach patient to sit close to pedals to avoid hyperextension of lumbar spine when driving is resumed. Issue long-handled shoehorn to facilitate dressing.

R–Bed rest. Place a firm plywood bedboard under mattress. Bend mattress at knee level over suitcase, and use bolster to elevate head and neck for semiseated bed reading posture, or obtain adjustable hospital bed.

I–Order lumbosacral corset. (See Fig. 63.)

E–Teach body mechanics to minimize low back stress, with emphasis on squatting rather than bending, and on proper techniques for lifting and for sitting. Instruct patient to stand with one foot on a 4- to 6-inch footstool while ironing and while preparing meals, washing dishes, etc.

S–Reassure the patient that the prognosis is favorable.

Comment: The patient suffered a strain to the lumbosacral area and a probable incomplete tear of an anulus fibrosus. This episode appears to be brief and self-limited, but present discomfort and future recurrences can be minimized with careful management.

CASE 12: Acute Lumbar Disk Herniation with L₅ Radiculopathy

A 34-year-old social worker has been aware of episodes of low back pain lasting one to five days for several years. Eight days prior to examination she developed a severe, diffuse low back pain while bending over to pull weeds in her garden. This pain abated somewhat after a week in bed, but a severe pain radiating down the right posterior thigh to the lateral calf and ankle ensued on arising from the toilet one day ago. Her past history and review of systems were not contributory.

Examination reveals a healthy-appearing young-middle-aged female who is in obvious pain when changing position. There is mild spasm of the paraspinal muscles with focal tenderness of the right erector spinae muscles at their origin overlying the right lumbosacral juncture. Tenderness on pressure over the spine of L_5 is also elicited. Straight leg raising is limited to 30 degrees on the right, 75 degrees on the left. The right medial hamstring reflex is slightly hypoactive. There is slight weakness of the long toe extensors and the anterior tibial muscle on the right. No sensory changes can be detected. Routine laboratory examinations and radiograms of the lumbar spine and pelvis are within normal limits. No EMG was done.

Assessment:

D–Acute lumbar disk protrusion with right L_5 radiculopathy

I–Minimal, associated with disk and nerve root trauma-

S–Probably L_5–S_1 disk and right L_5 root compression

C–Acute

O–None

R–Lumbar paraspinal muscle spasm

D–L_5 nerve root compression, right

Treatment:

M–Cold or warm compresses may be tried over the lumbar spine and areas of referred pain in the leg 20 to 30 minutes p.r.n. for pain relief.

E–Defer until pain subsides and neurological status stabilizes.

M–Bed rest

O–Instruct in grooming, feeding, self-care, and other activities to minimize back stress while in bed. (See Figs. 40 to 42.)

R–Bed rest on a firm mattress or mattress and bed board. Supine position with knee flexed and mild neck and dorsal spine flexion, if tolerated. Similar "hook" position for side lying. Use pillow between legs if needed to prevent aggravation of back pain by pelvic rotation as a consequence of traction from the weight of the leg. Avoid constipation. Transfer to bed-side commode or nearby toilet is preferable to using a bed pan for bowel movements in a male, and for both bowel and bladder evacuation in females. The toilet seat should be raised and, if possible, arm supports or grab bars provided.

I–Bed rest for at least two weeks. Neurological signs should be stable or receding toward normal and pain subsiding before beginning periods of sitting or standing. A lumbosacral corset should be fitted and worn for any activity out of bed. (See Fig. 63.) Sitting should be started in an armchair with a firm seat and back and maximum support to lumbar spine in 5- to 10-minute periods once, then twice daily, doubled daily as tolerated. (See Fig. 51.) Standing with one foot on a 4- to 6-inch stool for no more than 5 minutes after a short walk around bedroom. Showering (with assistance) in this position with back stabilized against shower wall can replace bed bath after standing position is tolerated.

E–Explain nature of disease, prognosis, and importance of compliance with regimen. Teach and reinforce proper spine position during movement in bed and during transfer. Instruct in basic body mechanics for lumbar spine problems.

S–Obtain adequate help at home to assist patient and care for family needs. Provide employer with estimate of return to part-time work in 8 to 12 weeks. Avoid sexual intercourse for three weeks and resume then only if neurological status is stable or improving.

Comment: The acute low back pain of disk trauma ("lumbago") following stressful activity often abates somewhat temporarily, with the onset of a further insult causing disk extrusion and radiculopathy ("sciatica"). The EMG in uncomplicated cases will show no abnormalities for about two weeks.

CASE 13: Chronic "Decompensated" Back

A 46-year-old salesman has had chronic moderate to severe low back pain for 15 months and has been unemployed and on disability for 9 months because of his pain. Ten years ago he developed acute low back pain while carrying his sample case. This led to hospitalization and a laminectomy for a lumbar disk herniation. He had persistent discomfort following his surgery and did not return to work until a few months after a favorable settlement of litigation over liability for his back problem was made two years after his surgery. He was never really well nor free of pain since his initial episode, but he has been able to work off and on as a salesman. The current exacerbation of his back pain he again attributes to a strain at work. He separated from his wife two months prior to this episode and had suffered severe recent financial reverses. He has been depressed and has mentioned suicide to friends more than once. He has had a prior history of duodenal ulcer, smokes 1½ packs of cigarettes per day and occasionally drinks excessively. He presently requires four Empirin with codeine #4, eight Tylenol tablets, and one to four Darvon 65 mg. tablets per day or pain relief, and two Dalmane tablets for sleep.

Examination reveals a depressed middle-aged male who dwells on his symptoms, and is somewhat dramatic in his movements when asked to bend forward or roll over. He has diffuse tenderness over the low back, a well-healed low midline lumbar incision, and focal "trigger" areas on deep palpation over the origins of both erector spinae muscles at the lumbosacral junctures, in the superior lateral aspect of the right quadratus lumborum, over the right sciatic outlet, and in the right subgluteus maximus trochanteric bursa at the distal and slightly posterior aspect of the right greater trochanter. Straight leg raising is limited to 60 degrees bilaterally. Lumbar motion is painful in all planes, especially on extension. Reflexes are physiological. Muscle testing is normal. There is an area of questionable hypalgesia on the lateral right calf. Routine laboratory studies, including an HLA-B27 typing, are unremarkable. Radiograms reveal moderate narrowing of the intervertebral spaces between L_4 and L_5 and L_5 and S_1. There is a 2 mm. anterior displacement of L_5 on S_1. Osteophytes are prominent both anteriorly and posteriorly from L_4–S_1, and there is marked sclerosis of the L_5–S_1 facet joints. The lamina of L5 is absent on the right. There is residual radiopaque material in the inferior subdural space. EMG's have repeatedly demonstrated patchy areas of old denervation in an L_5 distribution on the right.

Assessment:

D–Lumbar discogenic disease; old L_5 radiculopathy: bursitis, right subgluteus maximus and trochanteric bursae

I–None

S–L_4–S_1 disks and facet joints. Trigger areas in erector spinae bilaterally and right quadratus lumborum and gluteus maximus muscles

C–Chronic

O–History of peptic ulcer and alcoholism. Depression.

R–Tight lumbar fascia and hamstrings

D–Minimal anterior displacement of L_5 on S_1

Treatment:

M–Hot or cold packs 20 minutes p.r.n. prior to exercise and for pain relief.

Try ultrasound or diathermy over trigger areas in an attempt to raise pain threshold.

Vapo-coolant spray and, if unsuccessful, injections locally of 1 per cent lidocaine into muscle trigger area one to two times weekly should be tried. Injection of 5 mg. triamcinolone hexacetonide in 3 ml. 1 per cent lidocaine into the gluteus maximus bursa every two to four weeks for a maximum of four injections and then every two to four months p.r.n. for pain relief.

E–Begin pelvic tilts five times b.i.d. for one week. (See Fig. 35.) Add abdominal isometrics three times b.i.d., increasing to five times b.i.d. in the next week. (See Fig. 37.) Progress through low back exercise regimen in precise steps, adding a new exercise only when previous exercises have been successfully performed and shown to be well tolerated. *Reinforce success* in each exercise and in each increment in activity. (See Figs. 21, 25, 36, 38 and 39.)

M–Increase walking tolerances in specified increments at specified intervals, e.g., three walks around the bedroom four times each day, or walk three-fourths block and back twice daily this week, then a full block next week. For the next two weeks drive no more than 15 minutes without stopping to get out of car to perform pelvic tilts and partial deep knee bends. (See Figs. 35 and 38.)

O–Basic body mechanics to avoid low back stress during activities of daily living must be taught. Teach transfer techniques for bed to standing, standing to chair or toilet, and for entry and exit from automobiles. (See Figs. 40 to 42.) Provide a firm car seat support and teach close-to-pedal driving position.

Provide long-handled shoehorn, elastic shoe laces, elevated toilet seat with grab bars, and properly fitted armchair. (See Fig. 70.) Recreational activities and options should be explored as each level of improvement permits new opportunities. *Reinforce successes.*

R–Bed rest 10 to 12 hours per day with a midmorning and midafternoon one-hour nap. Use a firm mattress and a bedboard (minimum $\frac{1}{2}$" plywood). Teach hook side-lying posture and supine knee flexed position with bolster for leg supports, or obtain adjustable hospital bed.

I–Order lumbosacral corset and check to ensure proper fit. (See Fig. 63.) Teach patient technique for putting on corset with back supported by leaning against a wall.

E–Explain nature of discogenic process, problems of mechanical instability, and need for proper body mechanics and back protection methods as well as for progressive exercise regimens for patient. Identify patient's goals and perceptions and reconcile them with those of the therapeutic program. Prepare patient for a long course and only partial but definite improvement, consistent with realistic goals.

S–Determine the economic factors in the patient's life. Explore the exploitation of his "sick role" and the opportunities for him in reaching out to a "well role." Explain the "amplification phenomenon" in which *real symptoms become exaggerated by emotional factors.* Do not threaten his economic security by implying that his disability is not justifiable—if he chooses later to change his status, all well and good. Obtain consultation of a social worker and psychiatrist and closely coordinate efforts of all members of the health care team. Bring in family members and "significant others" for guidance and support. Discuss sexual problems frankly and offer concrete advice regarding positions and alternatives to intercourse. Begin a graduated drug detoxification program and coordinate with other pain-relieving modalities. If depression increases, consider antidepressant medication.

Comment: This patient is depressed as a consequence of his chronic pain and disability and socioeconomic failures. He now needs his pain to justify his new "career" as a person retired on disability. It is extremely difficult to sort out and identify a key treatable pathological focus in patients like this, and a multifaceted approach, preferably in a pain treatment center, usually offers the best chance for a favorable outcome—return to a satisfying life free of drugs, but not necessarily to gainful employment. Surgical consultation should be requested from an orthopedist or neurosurgeon familiar with the management of chronic back problems, but surgery is rarely indicated in these cases.

CASE 14: Osteoarthritis of the Hip

The patient is a 62-year-old female housewife who has had increasing difficulty with household activities and in engaging in her favorite recreation, golf, because of pain in her right hip. She first noted hip pain about five years ago. It had previously been intermittent but for the past six months it has been persistent, occasionally occurring at night. She has great discomfort on first arising from a sitting position and can walk only about one and a half blocks before severe pain precludes further ambulation.

Examination reveals mild restriction of motion of the right hip in all planes. Pain is elicited at the extremes of motion, and slight weakness of the hip abductors and extensors is detected on the right. There are no other significant abnormalities on examination. Radiograms show typical moderate advanced degenerative changes in the right hip. The laboratory reveals no abnormalities.

Assessment:

D–Osteoarthritis of the right hip
 I–±
S–Right hip
C–Chronic
O–Noncontributory
R–Lack of about 20 degrees in all planes of right hip motion
D–None

Treatment:

M–Trial of moist compresses for 20 minutes p.r.n. for pain relief. If no benefit, try diathermy 20 minutes, three times per week, for two weeks.

E–Active-assisted range of motion in all planes twice daily. Six-second isometrics to hip extensors and abductors twice daily. (See Figs. 48 and 49.) Advise concerning use of pool for range of motion therapy and general conditioning activities.

M–The patient is fitted for a cane and taught proper gait with cane in left hand.

O–Evaluate household activities to minimize unnecessary walking and standing. Provide patient with a long-handled shoehorn and a reacher to assist in picking up objects from the floor. Provide an elevated toilet seat and instruct patient to sit in firm, tall armchairs to facilitate transfer.

R–Ad lib.

 I–None

E–Patient should be taught to avoid excessive ambulation and prolonged standing, to select proper seating, and to understand the progressive nature of her hip disease. Discuss possible future surgery, the nature of the procedures, and the overall prognosis.

S–Discuss implications of restriction of physical activities as a consequence of disability. Discuss any problems with sexual relations.

Comment: This patient is approaching the day when a total hip replacement will become mandatory. Nonetheless, a well-balanced program in a compliant patient may postpone that day for worthwhile periods of time.

CASE 15: Osteoarthritis of Knee, Anserine Bursitis

A 62-year-old black woman has for several years had episodes of aching in the left knee after prolonged walking. For the past two months the pain has been almost constant when she has been on her feet, but largely relieved by rest. Stiffness of 10 to 15 minutes' duration is present in the morning and after prolonged sitting or lying. She has worked hard all her life, but does not recall any specific knee or other joint injury. Aside from occasional aching in her right shoulder and low back, she has had no other rheumatic complaints and has enjoyed good health. Aspirin gives partial relief. She has used a camphor liniment at bedtime for the past few weeks, and also a heating pad, both of which help reduce the aching in her knee.

On examination the patient appears moderately obese but in no distress except when bearing weight on the left knee. Her vital signs are normal. There is full range of motion in all joints, except for moderate restriction of all planes of motion in the lumbar spine. Both knees have slight varus deformities, more marked on the left. There is no redness, heat, or swelling about either knee. There is mild tenderness along the medial joint margin of the left knee, and palpable bony proliferations are present at the medial joint margins. There is slight medial and lateral collateral ligament instability, and stressing the medial collateral ligament is painful. The cruciate ligaments are intact. There is mild crepitation but no pain on compression of the patella during left knee flexion-extension. McMurray's sign is negative, but there is a grating sensation in the medial tibiofemoral compartment during this maneuver. There is exquisite tenderness elicited by thumb pressure over the anserine bursa area on the anteromedial aspect of the tibia about 1.0 cm. below the joint margin. The right quadriceps is slightly atrophied but has grade 5 strength on the manual muscle test. There are no clinical abnormalities of the right shoulder. Routine laboratory screening for rheumatic diseases is negative. X-rays reveal moderate narrowing of the medial tibiofemoral compartment of the right knee on the standing AP view. There is sclerosis of the medial tibiofemoral joint margins, with prominent osteophytes on the medial aspect of the tibiofemoral joint and on the intracondylar eminences. The lumbar spine shows evidence of moderate discogenic disease and anterior osteophyte formation. Shoulder radiograms are normal.

Assessment:

D–Osteoarthritis, left knee; anserine bursitis
 I–Mild
 S–Left knee
 C–Chronic with subacute exacerbation
 O–Obesity; probable periarthritis, right shoulder; lumbar osteo-
    arthritis
 R–None

D–Valgus deformity, slight collateral ligament instability

Treatment:

M–Continue superficial heat p.r.n.

E–Quadriceps isometrics, 6 seconds b.i.d. (See Fig. 50.) Range of motion, right knee and shoulder, once daily. (See Fig. 23.) Abdominal isometrics, pelvic tilts, and knee chest exercises once daily. (See Figs. 35 to 37.)

M–Patient should use cane in right hand to assist ambulation during exacerbations. Advise patient to avoid long walks, heavy loads, and walking on rough terrain, hills, or stairs.

O–Teach body mechanics and joint protection to minimize stress on shoulder, back, and knee. (See Figs. 40 to 42.) Have patient purchase proper foot-supporting walking oxfords for everyday use. Provide elevated toilet seat, grab bars, and properly fitted armchair. Provide a long-handled shoehorn and a reacher, to assist in picking up dropped objects. (See Figs. 70 and 71.) Have patient use a shopping cart in the market and a kitchen utility cart at home. Teach patient to arrange household and kitchen items so that she does not have to bend or climb or reach for bulky or heavy equipment.

R–Avoid unnecessary walking, and sit or lie down *before* pain is exacerbated.

I–A spiral knee cage may give some support and comfort for the right knee. A support stocking may be needed if dependent edema develops.

E–Explain degenerative arthritis and associated bursitis. Teach patient importance of minimizing joint stress. Reassure her regarding the local nature of her problem and the overall good prognosis if she complies with her regimen.

S–The patient is a housewife and not otherwise employed. Her family and economic situation are stable. She has maintained an active social and community life, which should be continued in the future.

Comment: This patient has developed osteoarthritis of the medial tibiofemoral compartment of the left knee, apparently secondary to constitutional varus deformities and associated greater weight-bearing stress on the medial than on the lateral tibiofemoral compartment. Her major focus of pain may well be in the anserine bursa, which is being stressed by the altered knee mechanics. A local steroid injection into the anserine bursa may greatly shorten the period of disability. An intra-articular steroid injection may also prove helpful if relief cannot be obtained with local measures, analgesics, or nonsteroidal anti-inflammatory drugs. Obesity is an aggravating factor. Her therapy, consisting of aspirin, superficial heat, and a liniment, is appropriate but has proved to be insufficient. Her back and shoulder are not a problem at present, but future trouble may be prevented by teaching proper body mechanics and joint protection.

CASE 16: Periarthritis, Chronic, Shoulder

A 54-year-old accountant developed persistent aching in the right shoulder following a weekend of household remodeling and painting chores. This episode had occurred four weeks previously. He has been in excellent health except for the shoulder problem. Examination at this times demonstrates a lack of 45 degrees of shoulder flexion and abduction and of 30 degrees of internal and external rotation. Mild to moderate pain is elicited at the extremes of motion and there is tenderness on direct pressure over the biceps groove. There is no discernible atrophy of the shoulder musculature. Muscle strength, when tested in a position of comfort, is normal, as is the remainder of the neurological examination. Radiograms of the neck and shoulder reveal no abnormalities.

Assessment:

D–Bicipital tendinitis with adhesive capsulitis
 I–1+
S–Right shoulder (glenohumeral)
C–Subacute–chronic
O–Noncontributory
R–Moderate
D–None

Treatment:

M–Moist compress 20 minutes every two to four hours, p.r.n.
 E–"Wall walking" for maximum flexion, followed by wand exercises for flexion and internal and external rotation, five repetitions of each exercise three times daily, after moist heat application. (See Figs. 14 to 16.)
M–Does not apply
O–Advise patient re long-handled tools to minimize overhead reaching when painting, to change wallet placement from left rear pocket to coat pocket, and to attach belt prior to putting on trousers.
R–Ad lib.
 I–Consider sling if symptoms exacerbate.
E–Teach patient to avoid sustained physical activity without proper conditioning and to appreciate value of pacing work assignments.
S–Does not apply.

Comment: Exercise regimen should be continued until full mobility is restored. When range of motion exercises are well tolerated, begin isometric exercise to the shoulder abductors and internal and external rotators. (See Fig. 46.)

CASE 17: Shoulder-Hand Syndrome

A 53-year-old male construction worker slipped on the job, fell, and suffered a minor strain of the right shoulder. He had mild discomfort in the shoulder for about two weeks but was able to continue working. Over the next two weeks the shoulder pain became increasingly severe and pain of equal intensity and swelling developed in the right hand and wrist. He has been treated with aspirin, codeine, and nonsteroidal anti-inflammatory drugs without benefit, and he has refused hot packs and exercise because they increase his discomfort. During the past four weeks he has not been able to use his right arm and there has been a progressive stiffening of the shoulder and hand. He has become quite despondent over his inability to get relief and to return to work.

Physical examination reveals a healthy-appearing middle-aged male with normal vital signs, who is obviously in discomfort and depressed. He is guarded in his verbal responses and partially resists attempts to examine his right arm because of pain. The right arm is carried in a partially flexed condition close to his body. The hand is mildly swollen, pale, cool, and moist. There is moderate restriction of motion of the wrist and of all finger joints, and any attempt at movement of these joints is painful. There is generalized tenderness, which is slightly accentuated on palpation over the PIP and MCP joints. There is a nodular thickening of the palmar fascia overlying the fourth MCP joint. The elbow is not tender and has a full range of motion; however, the shoulder is tender and is markedly restricted in both active and passive motion in all planes. The laboratory examination is entirely negative. Radiograms of the right shoulder, wrist, and hand show marked generalized demineralization and slight soft tissue swelling.

Assessment:
D–Shoulder-hand syndrome
 I–Mild
 S–Right shoulder, wrist, and hand
 C–Subacute
 O–Reactive depression
 R–Contractures of right shoulder, wrist, and hand
 D–Incipient nodular thickening of the palmar fascia

Treatment:
M–Cold compresses to shoulder, wrist, and hand for 20 minutes p.r.n. for pain relief—if tolerated.
E–Gentle active-assisted range of motion to affected areas. (See Figs. 2 to 6, 9 and 12 to 17.) Three sessions of one to three gentle stretches to each affected joint daily. When pain subsides sufficiently, increase vigor and frequency of stretches. Finally, add graduated isometric resistance and ultimately dynamic resistance exercises, utilizing weaving, sawing, sanding, and related functional activities. (See Figs. 43 to 46.) The key focus is on pain relief, then restoration of motion. If functional motion can be restored, some strengthening and increased endurance will result from usage alone but will be augmented by resistance exercises.
M–Not applicable

O–Functional training and adaptation for primarily unilateral hand activity by unaffected left hand until function begins to return to right hand. Encourage functional right-handed activities in ADL and with crafts and recreation as soon as tolerated to increase mobility and strength.

R–Not applicable

I–An arm sling and positioning hand splint for support during the active phase should be worn for pain relief and to minimize deformities. (See Table 5–1.) Spring wire splints may be needed to restore mobility when pain is controlled. (See Figs. 7 and 8.)

E–Reassure patient that the disorder is self-limited. Emphasize need for exercise to maintain motion and prevent permanent loss of function.

S–Arrange for financial support during period of disability. Refer for psychological counseling and consideration for antidepressant medications.

Comment: This middle-aged man has developed a very painful condition that has caused significant loss of motion and function in his right arm and threatens to destroy his ability to work. He suffers from a reactive depression, and it is also possible that a premorbid psychological state predisposed him to the autonomic derangement that characterizes the shoulder-hand syndrome. He is well into the course of this disorder and therefore may respond less well to stellate ganglion blocks or systemic steroids. Nonetheless, they should be tried in an attempt to control pain and interrupt this process. Intensive physical therapy to restore joint mobility is crucial but extremely difficult to implement if pain cannot be controlled. Of additional interest are the sparing of the elbow and the evidence of an early Dupuytren's contracture. The former is invariably found and the latter is commonly associated with the shoulder-hand syndrome.

CASE 18: Thoracic Outlet Syndrome

A 41-year-old housewife complains of a numb sensation in her hands, which is particularly troublesome on arising, especially when she sleeps supine with her hands above her head. It occasionally awakens her at night and is also noticeable when she engages in activities requiring overhead reaching, such as window washing, wall cleaning, and dusting high shelves. She has been aware of these symptoms for two years, but lately they have become more intense. The sensation of numbness may last for a few seconds to several minutes and appears to be relieved by shaking her hand to "improve the circulation." She has had no Raynaud's phenomenon and no other neurological, vascular, or musculoskeletal complaints. She has been in good health except for her intermittent numbness and feels no residual weakness or discomfort between episodes.

Examination reveals a moderately obese middle-aged woman with "round," slumping shoulders, a forward lordotic neck posture, and heavy, pendulous breasts. The scapulae are abducted and the pectoral muscles are shortened. There is no gross weakness of any muscle group, and there is no evidence of sensory, articular, or vascular dysfunction or insufficiency. Tinel and Phalen's tests for carpal tunnel syndrome are negative. The Adson maneuver for thoracic outlet obstruction, costoclavicular compression testing (shoulder hyperextension or "military bracing"), and pectoralis minor compression testing (hyperabduction and external rotation of the shoulder) all reveal slight diminution of the radial pulses bilaterally at the extreme position in each test, but no manifestations of numbness or of vascular insufficiency are elicited. The Allen test for distal radial and ulnar arterial insufficiency is normal. Routine laboratory studies, including screening for rheumatic diseases, are normal. Radiograms of the cervical spine show slight narrowing between C_5 and C_6, and an accentuated cervical lordotic curve. Hand, chest, and shoulder radiograms are normal, and there is no cervical rib. EMG and nerve conduction studies in both upper extremities, including the cervical paraspinal muscles, are normal.

Assessment:

D–Thoracic outlet syndrome, probable

 I–None

 S–Both upper extremities

 C–Chronic, recurrent

 O–Pendulous breasts, poor "sagging" neck-shoulder posture, tight pectorals and abducted scapulae

 R–Lordotic neck

 D–None

Treatment:

M–None

 E–Stretch pectoral muscles (5 to 10 stretches q.i.d.). (See Fig. 18.) Strengthen levator scapulae and upper trapezii (shoulder shrugs) and middle trapezii and rhomboids (scapular adduction isometrics and vertical "push-ups"). (See Fig. 19.) Do 10 shrugs and 10 vertical push-ups q.i.d. Continue these exercises q.i.d. until symptoms abate, then reduce to b.i.d. Strengthen cervical musculature. Six-second isometric contractions of neck flexors and extensors b.i.d. (See Fig. 47.)

M–Not applicable except re neck posture when driving

 O–Teach proper sitting posture—head up, shoulders back. (See Fig. 51.) Avoid chairs with arms too high, which push arms up and shorten pectorals, or too low, which encourage sagging of scapulae and shoulder stabilizers. Modify work habits to avoid prolonged overhead reaching. Use extended handles on mops or ladders when necessary to reach high inaccessible areas. Provide supporting bra with wide, padded shoulder straps.

R–Instruct patient to avoid putting hands over head while resting or sleeping.

I–None

E–Reinforce exercise and body mechanics instructions. Explain anatomical basis for treatment.

S–None

Comment: The patient has symptoms compatible with a thoracic outlet syndrome, but, as is often the case, objective confirmation is lacking. In the absence of evidence of irreversible vascular or neuromuscular impairment, a trial of conservative therapy is warranted before attempting an invasive diagnostic angiographic procedure or a surgical "exploration."

CASE 19: Painful Thumb (CMC Osteoarthritis vs. DeQuervain's Disease vs. Long Thumb Flexor Tenosynovitis)

A 57-year-old pharmacist complained of pain in his right thumb for six months. He first noted discomfort on grasping after one week of taking inventory, during which time he used his hands excessively. His thumb was quite painful for four days. There was no redness, heat, or swelling. Symptoms improved with rest and nonsteroidal anti-inflammatory drugs after a few days; however, it has remained difficult to open tight bottles, to type labels, and to perform household tasks requiring right hand grasp.

Examination reveals a "Heberden's" node on the left fourth finger attributable to an old injury, tenderness in the region of the right "snuff box" dorsally, but no tenderness or prominence of the first carpometacarpal joint on the dorsal or palmar surface (degenerative joint disease of the CMC unlikely). There is no "triggering" of the thumb and no crepitation on the palmar aspect of the first CMC or of the first metacarpophalangeal joints during active or passive thumb IP flexion (no flexor tenosynovitis). Tinel's sign was negative, and no muscle weakness not attributable to pain is detected. There is no muscle atrophy or sensory change in the hand or elsewhere (carpal tunnel syndrome unlikely). There was marked tenderness over the radial styloid and a suggestion of swelling just proximal and dorsal to the styloid. Ulnar deviation of the right wrist with the thumb flexed and grasped by the fingers produced sharp pain at the base of the right thumb—a positive Finkelstein's sign consistent with DeQuervain's disease. Radiograms of the hands revealed only a small osteophyte at the left fourth DIP joint. There were no laboratory abnormalities.

Assessment:
D–DeQuervain's disease
 I–Mild inflammatory reaction
 S–Tendon sheath of the right short thumb extensor
 C–Subacute–chronic
 O–None
 R–None
 D–None

Treatment:
M–Cold compresses for severe exacerbations
 E–None
M–Not relevant
 O–Review daily activities to find and minimize those causing thumb stress. Consider adaptive tools or modified methods or handles on existing tools.
 R–Avoid repeated or excessive stress to the right hand.
 I–Prescribe thumb-stabilizing splint, plastic, with free distal phalanx and moderate to marked restriction of thumb MP and CMC motion. (See Fig. 55.)
 E–Stress need to minimize thumb activities.
 S–Not relevant

Comment: The two disorders most easily confused in this case are DeQuervain's disease and osteoarthritis of the CMC joint of the thumb. Both these disorders may benefit from similar splinting. Local steroid injections must be precisely placed, e.g., along the radial styloid laterally for DeQuervain's disease and into the CMC joint for osteoarthritis. In refractory cases where surgical intervention is required, precise localization of the anatomical lesions is crucial.

CASE 20: Trigger Finger

A 63-year-old engineer has noted intermittent pain in his right fourth finger for four months. He is vigorous, plays golf and tennis, and does almost all of his home maintenance and gardening chores. He has had multiple minor traumas over the years in the course of daily activities and during his high school and college athletic programs but has suffered no major or recent unusual trauma. He has had an occasional low back pain but no arthritis and no other significant illness.

Physical examination reveals a moderately obese male in obvious good health. The significant findings are limited to the right hand. There is no skin or bony abnormality and no joint tenderness or swelling of the hand. There is slight crepitation and mild tenderness on pressure over the volar aspect of the right fifth MCP joint (at the distal palmar crease) during passive flexion and extension movements of that joint.

When the patient makes a forced grasp with the right hand followed by active extension of the fingers, there is a perceptible delay and then a jerky extension movement of the right fourth finger, which is associated with obvious discomfort.

Assessment:
D–Idiopathic tenosynovitis
 I–Minimal
 S–Flexor tendon, right fourth finger
 C–Chronic
 O–None
 R–"Trigger finger"
 D–None

Treatment:
M–None
 E–None
M–None
 O–Use built up handles for forced grasp activities. Pace work, chores, and other activities to minimize prolonged stress
 R–Not applicable
 I–If steroid injection is unsuccessful or refused, try a PIP splint to be worn during activities. (See Fig. 57.)
 E–Reinforce joint protection as above.
 S–None

Comment: These findings are typical of an idiopathic tenosynovitis of the fourth finger flexor tendon. Local steroid injections into the flexor tendon sheath will often induce a remission, but additional therapeutic measures may help prevent recurrences or provide an alternative to injections or surgical intervention.

OCCUPATIONAL THERAPY CLASS FOR INPATIENT RHEUMATOID ARTHRITIS PATIENTS*

by
Linda Kales, O.T.R.
Annette Swezey, M.S.P.H.

GOAL: To help patient participate actively in his or her management so that he or she may achieve the optimal benefits of the therapeutic program. To achieve maximal rehabilitation through the process, which allows as much patient participation as possible, stressing patient independence and quality of performance.

OBJECTIVES: Patient will be able to utilize inpatient occupational therapy hospital learning in home situation and life style.

Patient will be able to:
1. State ways to:
2. Practice techniques to:
   a. Prevent further impairment or deformity
   b. Maintain existing abilities
   c. Restore as much function as possible
   d. Achieve independence in activities of daily living (if necessary)
   e. Conserve energy

I. General Occupational Therapy Class *Primary Content Areas*
   A. Joint protection
   B. Energy conservation/work simplification
   C. Pacing
      1. Scheduling activities
      2. Priorities

---

*Developed for use on Rheumatology Rehabilitation Unit, 5 North, UCLA Hospital.

    D. Use of adaptive equipment

    E. Activities of daily living

II. Content Areas Which Interface with Other Professionals in Health Team

    A. Reinforce patient's understanding of disease process

    B. Reinforce patient's knowledge of relevant terminology

    C. Reinforce range of motion exercises and transfer techniques taught by Physical Therapist

    D. Augment patient's coping skills

    E. Team-teach with nurse (dietitian's consultation) a nutrition component for patients

    F. Education of family by all health team professionals whenever appropriate

    G. Reinforce proper use of medication by nurse in order to coordinate, when appropriate, analgesic medications with exercise periods

PRE-SESSION I   Individualized O.T. Evaluation and Orientation

SESSION I   Overview of O.T. Program

OBJECTIVES: Patient will be able: to discuss each day's schedule in hospital, role of O.T. in treatment of rheumatoid arthritis, and conservation of energy; to practice two methods of joint protection; to find community sources for adaptive equipment.

Content Areas	Teaching Materials and Methods	Evaluation Tools
Daily activities in hospital unit	Review daily activity schedule handout Group discussion Question and answer period	Prior to Session I initial evaluation on one-to-one basis
Conservation of energy Delegation of responsibility	Present conservation of energy handout Discussion of energy handout Question and answer period	Observation of patient's responses recorded in patient's medical chart
Joint Protection Rationale: to reduce pain, to protect and preserve joints	Discussion – Introduction Reinforcement by practice of position changes every 20 minutes Question and answer period Provided: felt tip pen to introduce, reinforce, and practice placing less stress on hand joints	*Return demonstrations
Splinting as a method for joint protection and rest	Introduction of hand splinting as a form of joint protection and joint rest Demonstrate two types of splints	Use of splints by specific patients after splint is made
Adaptive equipment Reasons for use of equipment: 1. Prevent further joint stress 2. Prevent pain 3. Conserve energy 4. Allow continuation or assumption of more responsibility for self-care	Community sources for individualized adaptive equipment presented	

*Return demonstration: have patient show O.T. what has been demonstrated by O.T. or other patients.

SESSION II   Management of Daily Activities

OBJECTIVES: Patient will be able to state routine of daily activities prior to hospitalization.
Patient will be able to problem-solve his and other patients' home activity schedules.
Patient will be able to give in his own words one reason for pacing his activities.
Patient will be able to state needs to balance rest and activity with level of disease activity.

Content Areas	Teaching Materials and Methods	Evaluation Tools
Home daily activities	Discussion in groups	Observation of participation of group and individuals in discussions and problem-solving
Balance between rest and activity	Problem-solving with activities written on easel as learning vehicle	
Pacing		
Reinforce first session	Handout of energy conservation of Session I reviewed	Observe patients' note taking, answers to questions in discussion period with regard to pacing
	Review important points of Session II with group input	Record patients' responses in medical chart
	Question and answer session	

SESSION III

OBJECTIVES: Principles and Practice of Hand Protection

Patients will be able to:

State two general physiological terms used in reference to the hand and arm.
Discuss the principles of how to use hands to avoid ulnar deviation.
Practice use of larger joints in hand activities.
Demonstrate ways to avoid static holding.

Content Area	Teaching Materials and Methods	Evaluation Tools
Hand physiology	Illustrations for physiology and terminology. Use Brattström, M: *Principles of Joint Protection in Chronic Rheumatic Disease*, Year Book, Chicago, 1975.	Patient able to draw correct lines to labels illustrating parts of hand anatomy
	Demonstration of aids and techniques	Observation of patient using book rack in hospital room
	Reading:	
	– Books on a rack	Return demonstration of how to use hands to avoid ulnar deviation
	– Use of rubber finger tip to turn pages	
	Writing:	Multiple choice test on terminology included in post-test
	– Use of felt-tip or built-up pen	
	– Stretch fingers every 10 to 15 minutes	
	– Electric typewriter/cassette recorder as alternatives	Various return demonstrations on joint protection methods
	Telephone:	
	– Use of pencil or stick for dialing	Observation of patient's participation written in medical chart
	– Pushbutton phone	
	– Alternate ears and hands frequently	
	– Talk for short periods of time	
	Doors/Drawers:	
	– Rubber doorknob extension	
	– Proper position to approach door handles	
	– Use of hip or side of body to close drawers	
	– Use of towel or webbing with loop on forearm to open refrigerator/oven/cupboard door	
	Faucets:	
	– Use of wooden tap turner (handout on how to construct)	
	– Dampened washcloth to facilitate grip	
	Keys: adapted key holder	
	Cards: card holder	
	Car door: opener	
	Jars: jar wrench, rubber pad, dampened washcloth	
	Plugs:	
	– Avoid plugging and unplugging by use of extension cords and on-off switch remote control set	

SESSION IV   Leisure

OBJECTIVES: Patient will be able to list two or more leisure activities which are generally recommended for patients with Rheumatoid Arthritis.
Patient will be able to transfer learning of hand joint protection to at least two activities which are considered recreational by discussing satisfactory alternative ways to "play".

Content Areas	Methods and Materials	Evaluation Tools
Types of leisure activities	Lecture plus discussion of problems and solutions to areas frequently involved in the following activities:	Orally listing recommended leisure activities
Indoors		
Outdoors	Painting and artwork: – Reinforce avoiding static holding – Reinforce building up handles on brushes	

Activity choices vary with disease activities	Embroidery/sewing:
	– Demonstration of one-handed loop on table top
	– Use of scissors discouraged, with rationale
	– Recommended hints:
	  Needle threader with large eyes on needles
	  Large-headed pins for less small pinching in hands
	  Magnet to pick up pins
	  Thread needle while still in pin cushion
	  Large yarn for embroidery	

	Crocheting/knitting: – Build up crochet hook or knitting needles to assist hand function of individual patients – Stretch fingers every 10 to 15 minutes	
	Music: – Suggest short periods, 15–30 minutes playing – Light touch electric piano or organ – Building up knobs of TV, radio, or stereo for joint protection	Return demonstration

Swimming a recommended activity:
– Suggest easy-to-remove suit for hand joint protection reinforcement
– Suggest heat pool to 90°F.

Golf, how it maintains range of motion but may be stressful to joints
– Suggestions:
Build up handles
Motorized cart or caddy
Appropriate time to golf

Question and answer periods relating new activity to previous discussions

Fishing and its problems:
– Suggestions:
Change position frequently
Prop up fishing pole
Build up handle of pole
Use of more rigid rod and easy action reels

Discussions

Yard work and the appropriate ways to garden. Relate to other joint protection discussions
– Suggestions:
Use long-handled tools
Use lightweight tools (children's tools)
Use lightweight power equipment
Raise gardening areas
Use sprinkler and soaker hose
Build up handles of gardening tools
Use stool to sit on if necessary in garden

O.T. multiple choice test

Discussion of activities not recommended and question and answer period:
– Tennis
– Basketball
– Archery
– Hiking on rough terrain
– Jogging
– Bicycling, bowling, dancing, yoga need individualized assessments

Observation of patient's response to suggestions about activities recorded in medical chart

SESSION V Work Simplification: Related to Kitchen and Home and Vocation

OBJECTIVES: Patient will be able to demonstrate three joint protection and work simplification techniques in the O.T. area kitchen.

Patient will be able to state two reasons for doing joint protection activities in the prescribed manner.

Content Areas	Methods and Materials	Evaluation Tools
Work simplification in relation to vocation	Introduction of film with philosophy of applying only what is pertinent to individual	
Energy Conservation	16 mm. color film: *The Handicapped Homemaker with Arthritis*	Observation of patients watching film
Philosophy of self-care when possible	Discuss independence	Observation of participation in group in discussion following film
	Reinforce practice of position change after twenty minutes of watching film	
	Discussion of film	
	Question and answer session	Return demonstration in O.T. kitchen area
		Pre-post multiple choice O.T. questionnaire

SESSION VI Work Simplification Related to Kitchen and Home

OBJECTIVES: See Section V Objectives

Content Areas	Materials and Methods	Evaluation Tools
Work simplification related to kitchen; home maintenance	Demonstration of some adaptive tools/methods in the kitchen which were in the Handicapped Homemaker film —Opening cans and jars and cartons —Demonstration of electric can opener —Wet cloth or Dycem® pad for opening jar tops —Pop-top cans: use end of knife or spoon —Milk cartons: use palms of hands —Avoid pull tab on cans: use electric can opener Reinforce principles of joint protection of hand with above examples. Demonstration of *stirring* in kitchen Suggestions: —Use lightweight bowls —Stabilize bowls with damp cloth or Dycem® pad underneath —Use flat bottom measuring spoons —Stir toward body, reinforce joint protection —Build up utensil handles with foam rubber —Use electric mixer or hand beater rather than fork Demonstration of *carrying*: —Rolling cart for heavy pans, utensils, and ingredients —Using two hands to lift —Double-handed pots —Using palms to lift from side or bottom of pot —Slide heavy objects on counter top	Return demonstration with reasons for using method suggested. O.T. multiple choice questionnaire Observations charted

SESSION VI (*continued*)   Work Simplification Related to Kitchen and Home

Content Areas	Materials and Methods	Evaluation Tools
Work simplification and joint protection	Carrying (continued) – Fill pan on stove from pitcher or spray hose – Use hoop apron with pockets to carry items – Cook in strainer to avoid draining	Return demonstration carrying and cutting food in kitchen area
	Demonstration of *cutting*: – Cutting board with suction cups, side and nails – Electric knife – Use rocker knife with two hands – Serrated knife – Parboil or cook vegetables before cutting – Use precooked frozen or dried vegetables to avoid cutting or peeling	
	Demonstration of *storage*: Suggestions and general rules: – Store things when they are first used, e.g., pots near stove within easy reach – Frequently used items within easy reach, in front portion of shelf – Store heavy items within easy reach, e.g., elbow level – Avoid buying large containers/jars – Store lightweight items higher up – Keep important appliances out on counter – Keep appliances plugged in and use on/off switch – *DON'T* stack bowls or cans – Keep shelves shallow, only 1 row deep – Use Rubbermaid pull-out shelves – Use lazy susan within easy reach to store – Hang utensils within easy reach of work area	Practice some of listed activities
	Handout: "Easy is the Name of the Game" for home reference and review	Problem-solving session relating to kitchen activities (See Session IX)

SESSION VII Work Simplification Related to Kitchen and Home Activities

OBJECTIVES: Patient will be able to name two work simplification methods which are efficient in energy conservation and will also protect small joints in hands.

Content Areas	Materials and Methods	Evaluation Tools
Work simplification and joint protection	Demonstration of: – Ironing – Dusting – Bedmaking – House cleaning – Kitchen efficiency – Clean up – Floor care – Laundry – Food protection	Return demonstration Observation of applying techniques learned in "class meal making"
	Reinforce by discussion hand joint protection in all above areas and use of large joints rather than small joints	O.T. multiple choice test
	Reinforce by discussion reason for energy conservation in above activities	

SESSION VIII Nutrition and Meal Preparation

OBJECTIVES: Patient will be able to plan meal in group using basic four food groups as criteria for balanced diet.
Patient will be able to interrelate with other patients to share task responsibilities.

Content Areas	Materials and Methods	Evaluation Tools
Basic Nutrition	Team-teaching with Nursing	
Overweight as stress on joints	Slide-cassette on nutrition (University of Michigan)	
Interpretation of fad diets	Arthritis Foundation handout on diet	
Sharing responsibilities	Discussion	Observation of patient's meal planning
	Group dynamics of meal planning	Observation of delegating responsibility
	—Group assigns specific tasks by individuals according to abilities and disabilities	Record observations of patient on chart

OCCUPATIONAL THERAPY CLASS 205

SESSION IX Problem Solving Session — Alternatives

OBJECTIVES: Patient will be able to relate in session two solutions to activities which have previously been a problem for him or her.
Patient will be able to demonstrate ability to participate in a group cooking activity.

Content Areas	Materials and Methods	Evaluation Tools
Review of problem-solving activities in the kitchen	Discussion and writing group problem-solving on easel with pad of newsprint and felt-tip pen in the format of problem activity and solution with methods for joint protection	Test on knowledge of disease and principles of joint protection
Review areas covered: — Grocery shopping — Opening cans — Opening jars — Opening and closing faucets — Peeling — Chopping — Carrying — Reaching — Handling pots and pans — Handling plates — Wringing out items — Opening and closing doors/drawers		Observation of practice of joint protection techniques in O.T.–P.T. area and patient's room
Practical kitchen activities	Application of meal planning, eating, and clean-up activities by group participation in eating "group-made" meal.	Observation of group dynamics Observation of ability to delegate responsibility

SESSIONS X AND XI   Personal Hygiene and Bathroom

OBJECTIVES: Patients will be able to demonstrate methods of joint protection and work simplification relating to personal hygiene tasks.

Content Areas	Materials and Methods	Evaluation Tools
Personal hygiene with joint protection	Hygiene demonstrations using patient's personal equipment when possible	
Work simplification	Teeth demonstration: Patients bring own toothbrush, toothpaste — Build up handle of toothbrush — Stabilize tube on washcloth — Squeeze paste with palm of hand — Electric toothbrush — Denture brush or cleaning tablet	Return demonstration of use of toothbrush and squeezing toothpaste
Range of motion exercises	Hair demonstration: Patients bring hairbrush and comb — Build up handle — Long-handled brush for severe loss of shoulder ROM and strength — Use large comb vs. small	Return demonstration, hair brushing
	Shampooing hair: — Use of rubber brush — Sit on stool, use portable shower head	Return demonstration
	Shaving: — Safety razor, build up handle — Electric razor or cream as alternative — Support arm if necessary	O.T. multiple choice test
	Nail care: — Emery board instead of scissors — Build up emery board — File for short periods of time — Suction brush for cleaning — Nail clippers, cut after wetting to soften nails	

Deodorant:
– Roll-on preferred
– Lever handle for spray cans

Observation of practice in hospital room by nurses charting

Washing:
– Wash mitt with pocket for soap
– Avoid wringing of washcloth, drip-dry over faucet
– Long bath sponge
– Body sponge
– Soap-on-a-rope
– Oversize bath towel or terry robe for drying

Return demonstration, face washing in patient's room

Tub/Shower:
– Method of transfer
– Bench/chair
– Detachable hose
– Grab bars/safety rails
– Faucets, lever handles or use of washcloth to turn
– Organizer or shelf
– Rubber bath mat inside
– Non-skid rug

Observation of practice of new methods in use of shower or tub on hospital unit

Toilet:
– Elevated seat
– Grab bars
– Sponge for cleaning
– Bidet

Above charted by O.T.

Sink area:
– Organize hygiene aids
– Sit to avoid fatigue
– Rest elbow on counter tops

Discussion of problem areas

SESSION XII   Dressing

OBJECTIVE: Patient will be able to select relevant dressing assistive devices to demonstrate principles of joint protection and philosophy of self-help.

Content Areas	Materials and Methods	Evaluation Tools
Joint Protection	Demonstration of putting on bra: —bra strap protectors —use of powder —hook bra in front and swing around	
Assistive Devices	Demonstration of buttoning: —various types of hooks —practice session with hooks —large buttons preferred	Return demonstration
	Demonstration of zippers: —zippers used with ring or yarn loop—if in the back use long handle or ring with dressing stick —cup hook on dowel	
	Demonstration of shoes: —Velcro closures —well-fitting slip-ons —introduce reasons for in-depth shoes —long shoe horn —elastic laces —long dressing stick —support foot on stool	Patient Ed. General Knowledge Test O.T. problem-solving multiple choice quiz

Demonstration of putting on
stockings:
– sock cone
– dressing stick
– cloth loops
– rub foot on foam pad for friction
– buy larger size

Discussion of neck ties:
– pre-knotted neckties
– loosen to remove and pull overhead

Demonstration of putting on skirt
or trousers:
– place loop on waistband

Demonstration of putting on belt
on skirt or trousers by putting belt
around prior to putting on skirt or
trousers

SESSION XIII

OBJECTIVES:

Review of O.T. Class

Patient will be able to have any misconceptions relating to patient questionnaire clarified.
Patient will be able to have concepts of energy conservation and joint protection
reinforced before leaving hospital setting.

Content Areas	Materials and Methods	Evaluation Tools
General review of all content areas	Post-test feedback General rap Question and answer session	General test of patients' knowledge of RA Discharge evaluation

O.T. MULTIPLE CHOICE QUESTIONNAIRE FOR PATIENTS*

Dear Patients:
Please check what you feel are the best solutions. Do not be concerned if you are not sure of your answers as we will be going over the solutions shortly. There can be *more than* ONE GOOD SOLUTION.

1. Mrs. Smith (a patient with mildly active R.A.) drove her car to the market expecting to pick up a few items for dinner that night; she had already done her "big" marketing with her neighbor who always helped carry things in the house for her. In the market Mrs. Smith was hungry and things really looked delicious to her. Before she knew it, the cart was half full. When it was check-out time at the market, should she:

    _____a. Request special light packaging?
    _____b. Try to carry a full load to save trips back and forth from her car to the garage?
    _____c. Put back all but her necessary groceries?
    _____d. Leave the groceries packed and pick them up when her family is available?

2. Mr. Morse has R.A. and he enjoys settling down for the evening for a good TV movie. He places his TV tray by his side with a drink (Coke?) and some peanuts at his side so he will not have to get up and down for the next two hours. Which of the following would be good advice for him?

    _____a. He should not set himself up so that he will not move for two hours.
    _____b. He should leave his peanuts in the kitchen or in a place so that he will have to move during the ads.
    _____c. He should place a pillow under his knees so that they can be comfortable while he watches TV.
    _____d. He should place the telephone next to him also so that he will not constantly have to get up to answer it.

3. Mrs. Martin, a patient with rheumatoid arthritis, has always done her own ironing. She's told her family, "That's one thing the family is not going to be able to do for me." Her hands are starting to deviate "ulnarly" and many times her knees just plain hurt. How should she work on ironing?

    _____a. Sit up on a high stool with a back and foot rest.
    _____b. Use lightweight iron.
    _____c. Iron a few items at a time.
    _____d. Finish items as quickly as possible.

4. Mrs. Verité is visiting a friend and feels very uncomfortable sitting in her friend's new low couch. She ponders about how to respond to her "new" aches and remembers that she had left her foam cushion (which she used at the dentist's) in the car. Which would you choose for Mrs. Verité's approach to the problem?

---

*Developed for use in Rheumatology Unit, 5 North, UCLA Hospital, by Annette M. Swezey, M.S.P.H. Director of Arthritis Patient Education, UCLA.

_____a. Suffer in the low chair and not get her foam cushion.

_____b. Ask her friend to get her foam cushion from the car.

_____c. Ask her friend if she might have a straight chair as she feels more comfortable sitting that way.

Remember, there may be *more than* ONE *correct solution.*

5. Mr. Jones has always enjoyed sharing his vegetable garden with his neighbors. This year everyone has said for him not to bother, as his R.A. in his hip was in "a flare." However, he carefully planted, sitting on a stool in the garden, and is now enjoying the fruits of his labors. He is eager to share his various vegetables. Should he:

_____a. Allow his neighbors to pick their own?

_____b. Do his own garden harvest so that he will have vegetables to give his neighbors and relatives as usual?

_____c. Arrange a special "harvest day" once a week in which all his neighbors can participate while he supervises?

6. Mrs. Fuller loved to brush and comb her long pageboy hairdo; however, she was finding it more and more difficult to accomplish this activity. She was feeling frustrated. She had originally decided to cut her hair short, but kept postponing it. One day when she had a doctor's appointment, he suggested that she needed some exercises to make sure that her shoulder joints routinely went through a necessary range of motion. The O.T. recommended a long-handled comb and hairbrush in order to exercise range of motion in her shoulder routinely as she combed her pageboy.

_____a. Do you think that the O.T.'s solution made the exercise program convenient?   Yes _____   No _____

_____b. Do you think that short hair was a better solution?
                                    Yes _____   No _____

7. Hearing Mr. Ermin singing in his *shower* was as familiar an early morning sound in his house as that of the birds chirping in the trees nearby; however, he was constantly feeling weak and as if his knees would not hold him. He really didn't know what to do, as the thought of getting *stuck in the bathtub* seemed an even worse consequence than the feeling of weakness. For Mr. Ermin which do you think is safest:

_____a. Sitting on a bath bench in the shower?

_____b. Using a bathtub?

_____c. Leaning against the shower wall whenever he felt weak?

8. Mr. Adams was a bartender. He had his R. A. disease in good control but when he worked very hard his hands would swell from opening and closing all the necessary bottles and jars. A few things he could do to help his problem and protect his joints are:

_____a. Use a Zim jar opener.

_____b. Ask a waiter to open the bottles ahead of time and keep bottles loosely closed.

_____c. Pour large amounts of liquid into easy-to-open large bottles.

9. Mrs. Ramirez is her husband's bowling partner and she feels that it's an important activity which they share. The league meets once a week. She bowls five games and is very stiff and swollen the next day; however, she claims that it's worth it. Which of the ideas below allow for her continued sharing of bowling and not feeling poorly the next day?

_____ a. Try bowling only one game.
_____ b. Become the scorekeeper.
_____ c. Increase her medication so that it's working at the bowling hour.
_____ d. Stop going with her husband to the game.
_____ e. Bowl more so that she will get used to it and keep in bowling condition.

10. Mary McDougal's twin sons, who are five years old, love to make cookies with her as an afternoon activity. Mary, who has R.A., has trouble *stirring* the cookie dough. She does not like to use her electric mixer with the boys involved in "tasting" the dough to see if it's good. Her solution to this problem should be: (You can choose more than one correct answer.)

_____ a. Not making cookies with her sons.
_____ b. Building up with foam rubber the large spoon handle she uses to stir the cookie dough.
_____ c. Having the children take turns stirring the dough and finishing the stirring herself when it gets too stiff for them.
_____ d. Using a cookie dough recipe that can be kneaded with the palms of her hands and her children's hands too.

BIBLIOGRAPHY

1. Wood, P. H. N.: Classification of impairments and handicaps. World Health Organization. International Conference for the 9th Revision of the International Classification of Diseases. Geneva, September-October, 1975.
2. U.S. House of Representatives, Subcommittee on Social Security of the Committee on Ways and Means. *Disability Insurance — Legislative Issue Paper*. U.S. Government Printing Office, May 17, 1976. WMCP:94-132.
3. The Committee on Medical Rating of Physical Impairment: A guide to the evaluation of permanent impairment of the extremities and back. JAMA, Special Edition, Feb. 15, 1958.
4. Krusen, F. H., Kottke, F. J., Ellwood, P. M., eds.: *Handbook of Physical Medicine and Rehabilitation*. 2nd Ed. Philadelphia: W. B. Saunders Co., 1971.
5. Nuki, G., Brooks, R., Buchanan, W. W.: The economics of arthritis. Bull. Rheum. Dis., *23* (8–9):726, Series 1972–1973.
6. Wood, P. H. N., ed.: *The Challenge of Arthritis and Rheumatism*. London: The British League Against Rheumatism, 1977.
7. The Arthritis Foundation 1975 Annual Report. New York: The Arthritis Foundation, n.d. P. 2.
8. U.S. Congress, Department of Health, Education and Welfare. National Commission on Arthritis and Related Musculoskeletal Diseases. *Arthritis: Out of the Maze. Volume 1: The Arthritis Plan*. April, 1976. Publication No. NIH 76-1150.
9. Heather, A. J.: A two-year follow-up study of the patients admitted to the Rehabilitation Center of the Hospital of the University of Pennsylvania. Am. J. Phys. Med., *37* (5):237, Oct. 1958.
10. Robinson, H. S.: The cost of rehabilitation in rheumatic disease. J. Chronic Dis., *8*:713, Dec. 1958.
11. Goldman, R.: Finding jobs for arthritis patients. J. Rehabil., *25*:21, 1959.
12. Manheimer, R. H.: Arthritics in competitive employment. An eight-year experience. Arch. Environ. Health. (Chic.), *4*:495, May 1962.
13. Dixon, A. St. J., ed.: *Progress in Clinical Rheumatology*. Volume 1. London: J. & A. Churchill, 1965.
14. Katz, S., Vignos, P. J., Jr., Moskowitz, R. W., et al.: Comprehensive outpatient care in rheumatoid arthritis. A controlled study. JAMA, *206*:1249, Nov. 1968.
15. Karten, I.: Should your hospital have an arthritis midway house? Hospital Practice, *4*:66, Jul. 1969.
16. Harris, R.: "Chapter 19. Rehabilitation," *in* S. Licht, ed., *Arthritis and Physical Medicine*. Baltimore: Waverly Press, 1969. P. 458.
17. Duff, I. F., Carpenter, J. O., and Neukom, J. E.: Comprehensive management of patients with rheumatoid arthritis. Some results of the regional arthritis control program in Michigan. Arthritis Rheum., *17* (5):635, 1974.
18. Vignos, P. J., Jr., et al.: Comprehensive care and psycho-social factors in rehabilitation in chronic rheumatoid arthritis: a controlled study. J. Chronic Dis., *25*:457, Aug. 1972.

19. Acheson, R. M., Crago, A., Weinerman, È. R.: New Haven survey of joint diseases. Institutional and social care for the arthritic. J. Chronic Dis., *23*:843, May 1971.

20. Robinson, H. S.: "Prognosis: Return to work — Arthritis," *in* G. E. Ehrlich, ed., *Total Management of the Arthritic Patient.* Philadelphia: J. B. Lippincott Co., 1973. P. 183.

21. Nuki, G., Brooks, R., Buchanan, W. W.: *Bulletin on Rheumatic Diseases and Disability Insurance.* Legislative issue paper prepared by the staff on the Subcommittee on Social Security. Washington: U.S. Government Printing Office, May 1976. P. 28.

22. Ehrlich, G. E.: Rheumatic diseases in industry. Penn. Med., *72*:65, 1969.

23. Acker, M.: Vocational rehabilitation of the rheumatoid arthritic. J. Rehabil., *23*:12, 1957.

24. Karten, I., Lee, M., McEwen, C.: Rheumatoid arthritis: five-year study of rehabilitation. Arch. Phys. Med. Rehabil., *54*:120, Mar. 1973.

25. Scorzelli, J. F., Goldthwait, J. C., Myers, J. S.: *Rehabilitation and the arthritic client.* A report on the seminar held June 11, 1976, Robert Breck Brigham Hospital, Boston, Mass. Northeastern University Rehabilitation Counseling Program, Oct. 1976.

26. Goldthwait, J. C.: "Chapter IV. Bone, joint, and muscle disorders," *in* J. S. Myers, ed., *An Orientation to Chronic Disease and Disability.* New York: Macmillan, 1965.

27. Manheimer, R. H., Acker, M.: "Back to work" program for physically handicapped arthritics. J. Chronic Dis., *5*:770, June 1957.

28. Robinson, H. S., Walters, K.: Return to work after treatment of rheumatoid arthritis. Can. Med. Assoc. J., *105*:166, July 1971.

29. Goldstein, D. H., et al.: Second conference on rheumatic diseases in industry. Arch. Environ. Health, *4* (5):487, 1962.

30. California State Department of Rehabilitation. *Rehabilitation Services Manual, Section 132210.* Sacramento, CA. n.d.

31. Laurie, G.: *Housing and Home Services for the Disabled.* New York: Harper & Row, 1977. Pp. 77, 389–415.

32. California Department of Administrative Services, Office of Administrative Hearings. *California Administrative Code Title 22, Social Security Division 5, Licensing and Certification of Health Facilities and Referral Agencies.* Sacramento, CA. n.d.

33. Sokoloff, L.: *The Biology of Degenerative Joint Disease.* Chicago: The University of Chicago Press, 1969. P. 77.

34. Lawrence, J. S.: "Chapter 17. Climate and arthritis," *in* S. Licht, ed., *Arthritis and Physical Medicine.* Baltimore: Waverly Press, 1969. P. 440.

35. Lee, P., et al.: The etiology and pathogenesis of osteoarthrosis: a review. Semin. Arthritis Rheum., *3*:189, Spring 1974.

36. Radin, E. L.: Mechanical aspects of osteoarthrosis. Bull. Rheum. Dis., *26* (7):862, 1975–1976 series.

37. Lawrence, J. S., DeGraaff, R., Laine, V. A. I.: "Chapter 11. Degenerative joint disease in random samples and occupational groups," *in* J. H. Kellgren, ed., *Epidemiology of Chronic Rheumatism.* Volume 1. Oxford: Blackwell Scientific Publications, 1963. P. 98.

38. Kellgren, J. H.: Osteoarthrosis in patients and populations. Br. Med. J., *5243*:1–6, July 1961.

39. Leviton, G. L.: "Professional-client relations in a rehabilitation hospital setting," *in* W. S. Neff, ed., *Rehabilitation Psychology.* Washington, D.C.: American Psychological Association, Inc., 1971. P. 215.

40. Vineberg, S. E.: "Psychologists in rehabilitation — manpower and training," *in* W. S. Neff, ed., *Rehabilitation Psychology.* Washington, D.C.: American Psychiatric Association, Inc., 1971. P. 287.

41. Reed, J. W., Harvey, J. C.: Rehabilitating the chronically ill: a method for evaluating the functional capacity of ambulatory patients. Geriatrics, *19*:87, Feb. 1964.

42. Keith, R. A.: The comprehensive rehabilitation center as rehabilitation model. Inquiry, *8*:22, Sep. 1971.

43. Halstead, L. S.: Team care in chronic illness. A critical review of the literature of the past 25 years. Arch. Phys. Med. Rehabil., *57*:507, Academy Issue, Nov. 1976.

44. Kliment, S. A.: *Into the Mainstream — A Syllabus for a Barrier-Free Environment.* U. S.

Department of Health, Education and Welfare, Rehabilitation Services Administration. The American Institutes of Architects, Social and Rehabilitation Services, 1975. P. 26.

45. Erickson, E. R., Pedersen, E.: Design criteria for a rehabilitation unit. Hospitals, *39*:53, Mar. 1965.

46. Boyle, R. W.: "Chapter 9. The therapeutic gymnasium," *in* S. Licht, ed., *Therapeutic Exercise.* New Haven: Elizabeth Licht, 1961. P. 257.

47. Stewart, J. B.: "Chapter 10. Exercises in water," *in* S. Licht, ed., *Therapeutic Exercises.* 2nd Ed. Baltimore: Waverly Press, 1965. P. 285.

48. Huskisson, E. C.: Measurement in rehabilitation. Rheum. Rehabil., *15* (3):132, 1976.

49. Goodwill, C. J.: Introduction: Methods available so far. From Symposium on measurement in rehabilitation. Rheum. Rehabil., *15*:161, 1976.

50. Lee, P., et al.: Evaluation of a functional index in rheumatoid arthritis. Scand. J. Rheum., *2*:71, 1973.

51. Taylor, D.: A table for the degree of involvement in chronic arthritis. Can. M. A. J., *36*:608, June 1937.

52. Scranton, J., Fogel, M. L., Erdman, W. J., 2nd: Evaluation of functional levels of patients during and following rehabilitation. Arch. Phys. Med., *51*:1, Jan. 1970.

53. Ehrlich, G. E.: "Appendix A. Assessment of Function," *in* G. E. Ehrlich, ed., *Total Management of the Arthritic Patient.* Philadelphia: J. B. Lippincott Co., 1973. P. 233.

54. Ehrlich, G. E.: "Functional Assessment," *in* G. E. Ehrlich, ed., *Total Management of the Arthritic Patient.* Philadelphia: J. B. Lippincott, 1973. P. 247.

55. Haataja, M.: Evaluation of the activity of rheumatoid arthritis. Scand. J. Rheum., *4* (Suppl. 7):3, 1975.

56. Swanson, A. B., Mays, J. D., Yamauchi, Y.: A rheumatoid arthritis evaluation record for the upper extremity. Surg. Clin. N. Amer., *48*:1003, Oct. 1968.

57. MacBain, K. P.: Assessment of function in the rheumatoid hand. Can. J. Occup. Ther., *37*:95, Autumn 1970.

58. Treuhaft, P. S., Lewis, M. R., McCarty, D. J.: A rapid method for evaluating the structure and function of the rheumatoid hand. Arthritis Rheum., *14*:75, Jan.–Feb. 1971.

59. Jebsen, R. H., Taylor, N., Trieschmann, R. B., et al.: An objective and standardized test of hand function. Arch. Phys. Med., *50*:311, June 1969.

60. Robinson, H. S., et al.: Functional results of excisional arthroplasty for the rheumatoid hand. Can. M. A. J., *108*:1495, June 1973.

61. Carroll, D.: A quantitative test of upper extremity function. J. Chronic Dis., *18*:479, May 1965.

62. Dworecka, F. F., Challenor, Y., Spector, P., et al.: A practical approach to the evaluation of rheumatoid hand deformity. Amer. J. Orthop. Surg., *10*:96, Apr. 1968.

63. Willkens, R. F., Gleichert, J. E., Gade, E. T.: Proximal interphalangeal joint measurement by arthrocircameter. Ann. Rheum. Dis., *32*:585, Nov. 1973.

64. Goldie, I. F., Gunterberg, B., Jacobson, C.: Foot volumetry as an objective test of the effect of antiphlogistic drugs in ankle sprains. A preliminary study. Rheum. Rehabil., *13* (4):204, Nov. 1974.

65. Smyth, C. J., Velayos, E. E., Hlad, C. J., Jr.: A method for measuring swelling of hands and feet. I. Normal variations and applications in inflammatory joint diseases. Acta Rheum. Scand., *9*:293, 1963.

66. Mikulic, M. A., Griffith, R. N., Jebsen, R. H.: Clinical applications of a standardized mobility test. Arch. Phys. Med. Rehabil., *57*:143, Mar. 1976.

67. Jebsen, R. H., Trieschmann, R. B., Mikulic, M. A., et al.: Measurement of time in a standardized test of patient mobility. Arch. Phys. Med. Rehabil., *51*:170, Mar. 1970.

68. Katz, S., Ford, A. B., Moskowitz, R. W., et al.: Studies of illness in the aged. The index of ADL: a standardized measure of biological and psychosocial function. JAMA, *185*:914, Sept. 1963.

69. The Joint Committee of the Medical Research Council and Nuffield Foundation on Clinical Trials of Cortisone, A.C.T.H., and Other Therapeutic Measures in

Chronic Rheumatic Diseases: A comparison of cortisone and aspirin in the treatment of early cases of rheumatoid arthritis. Br. Med. J., *1*:1223, 1954.

70. Sarno, J. E., Sarno, M. T., Levita, E.: The functional life scale. Arch. Phys. Med. Rehabil., *54*:214, May 1973.

71. Crewe, N. M., Athelstan, G. T., Meadows, G. K.: Vocational diagnosis through assessment of functional limitations. Arch. Phys. Med. Rehabil., *56*:513, Dec. 1975.

72. Mahoney, F. I., Barthel, D. W.: "Functional evaluation: the Barthel Index," *in* D. G. Carrol, ed., *Rehabilitation*. Baltimore: Baltimore City Medical Society, 1965. P. 61.

73. Gersten, J. W., Ager, C., Anderson, K., et al.: Relation of muscle strength and range of motion to activities of daily living. Arch. Phys. Med. Rehabil., *51*:137, Mar. 1970.

74. Granger, C. V.: *A Monograph: A System for Management of Selected Data in Medical Rehabilitation*. Boston: Tufts University, 1973.

75. Granger, C. V., Greer, D. S.: Functional status measurement and medical rehabilitation outcomes. Arch. Phys. Med. Rehabil., *57* (3):103, 1976.

76. Convery, F. R., et al.: A functional assessment of polyarticular disability. The Division of Orthopaedics and Rehabilitation, University of California, San Diego. Unpublished data, January, 1976.

77. Willard, H. S., Spackman, C. S., eds.: *Occupation Therapy*. 4th Ed. Philadelphia: J. B. Lippincott Co., 1971. P. 219.

78. Robinson, H. S., Bashall, D. A.: "Functional assessment," *in* G. E. Ehrlich, ed., *Total Management of the Arthritic Patient*. Philadelphia: J. B. Lippincott Co., 1973. P. 241.

79. Ehrlich, G. E., ed.: *Total Management of the Arthritic Patient*. Philadelphia: J. B. Lippincott Co., 1973.

80. Steinbrocker, O., Traeger, C. H., Batterman, R. C.: Therapeutic criteria in rheumatoid arthritis. JAMA, *140*:659, June 1949.

81. Schoening, H. A., Anderegg, L., Bergstrom, D., et al.: Numerical scoring of self-care status of patients. Arch. Phys. Med., *46*:689, Oct. 1965.

82. Lowman, E. W.: Rehabilitation of the rheumatoid cripple: a five-year study. Arthritis Rheum., *1*:38, Feb. 1958.

83. Dinsdale, S. M., Mossman, P. L., Sullickson, G., Jr., et al.: The problem-oriented medical record in rehabilitation. Arch. Phys. Med. Rehabil., *51*:488, Aug. 1970.

84. MacBain, K. P., Hill, R. H.: A functional assessment for juvenile reheumatoid arthritis. Amer. J. Occup. Ther., *27*:326, Sept. 1973.

85. Eberl, D. R., et al.: Repeatability and objectivity of various measurements in rheumatoid arthritis: a comparative study. Arthritis Rheum., *19*:1278, Nov.–Dec. 1976.

86. Bäcklund, L., Tiselius, P.: Objective measurement of joint stiffness in rheumatoid arthritis. Acta Rheum. Scand., *13*:275, 1967.

87. Fries, J. F., Hess, E. V., Klinenberg, J.: A standard database for rheumatic diseases. Arthritis Rheum., *17*:327, May–June 1974.

88. Kelman, H. R., Willner, A.: Problems in measurement and evaluation of rehabilitation. Arch. Phys. Med., *43*:172, Apr. 1962.

89. Hess, E. V.: A uniform database for rheumatic diseases. Prepared by the Computer Committee of the Amer. Rheum. Assoc. Arthritis Rheum., *19*:645, May–June 1976.

90. Rancho Los Amigos Hospital Physical Therapy Department: *Guide for Treatment of Rheumatoid Arthritis*. Modification of the functional classification used by the American Rheumatism Association. January, 1969. P. 19.

91. Smythe, H. A.: Assessment of Joint Disease. Toronto, January, 1975. P. 10. Unpublished data.

92. Moskowitz, E., McCann, C. B.: Classification of disability in the chronically ill and aging. J. Chronic Dis., *5*:342, Mar. 1957.

93. Redford, J. B.: "Chapter 1. Classification of rheumatic diseases," *in* S. Licht, ed., *Arthritis and Physical Medicine*. Baltimore: Waverly Press, 1969. P. 1.

94. Zung, W. W. K.: A self-rating depression scale. Arch. Gen. Psychiat., *12*:63, 1965.

95. Zung, W. W. K., Wonnacott, T. H.: Treatment prediction in depression using a self-rating scale. Biol. Psychiat., *2*:321, Oct. 1970.

96. Rutter, B. M.: Measurement of psychological factors in chronic illness. Rheum. Rehabil., *15*:174, 1976.

97. Geertsen, H. R., Gray, R. M., Ward, J. R.: Patient non-compliance within the context of seeking medical care for arthritis. J. Chronic Dis., *26*:689, Nov. 1973.

98. Bogdonoff, M. D., Nichols, C. R.: Perspectives of chronic illness. JAMA, *174*:104, 1960.

99. Duthie, J. J. R., Thompson, M., Weir, M. M., Fletcher, W. B.: Medical and social aspects of the treatment of rheumatoid arthritis with special reference to factors affecting prognosis. Ann. Rheum. Dis., *14*:133, June 1955.

100. Nachemson, A.: Physiotherapy for low back pain patients. Scand. J. Rehabil. Med., *1* (2):85, 1969.

101. Schoening, H. A., Iverson, I. A.: The Kenny Self-Care Evaluation. *A numerical measure of independence in activities of daily living.* Minneapolis: Kenny Rehabilitation Institute, The American Rehabilitation Foundation, 1965.

102. Lee, P., Kennedy, A. C., Anderson, J., et al.: Benefits of hospitalization in rheumatoid arthritis. J. Med., New Series, *43*:205, Apr. 1974.

103. Mills, J. A., Pinals, R. S., Ropes, M. W., et al.: Value of bed rest in patients with rheumatoid arthritis. N. Engl. J. Med., *284*:453, Mar. 1971.

104. Partridge, R. E., Duthie, J. J.: Controlled trial of the effect of complete immobilization of the joints in rheumatoid arthritis. Ann. Rheum. Dis., *22*:91, 1963.

105. Perkins, G.: Rest and Movement. (Robert Jones Lecture) J. Bone Joint Surg., *35B*:521, Nov. 1953.

106. Kottke, F. J.: The effects of limitation of activity upon the human body. JAMA, *196* (10):825, 1966.

107. Cooper, R. R.: Alterations during immobilization and regeneration of skeletal muscle in cats. J. Bone Joint Surg., *54A*:919, July 1972.

108. Gault, S. J., Spyker, M. J.: Beneficial effect of immobilization of joints in rheumatoid and related arthritides: a splint study using sequential analysis. Arthritis Rheum., *12*:34, Feb. 1969.

109. Harris, R., Copp, E. P.: Immobilization of the knee joint in rheumatoid arthritis. Ann. Rheum. Dis., *21*:353, Dec. 1962.

110. Enneking, W. F., Horowitz, M.: The intra-articular effects of immobilization on the human knee. J. Bone Joint Surg., *54A*:973, July 1972.

111. Kamenetz, H. L.: "Chapter 15. Massage, manipulation and traction," *in* S. Licht, ed., *Arthritis and Physical Medicine.* Baltimore: Waverly Press, 1969. Pp. 394, 407, 408.

112. Lucas, M.: The place of physiotherapy in the management of lumbar disc lesions. Physiotherapy, *50*:289, Sept. 1964.

113. Watkins, R. A., Robinson, D.: *Joint Preservation Techniques for Patients with Rheumatoid Arthritis.* Chicago: Northwestern University, 1974. P. 16.

114. Sinclair, J. D.: "Exercise in pulmonary disease," *in* S. Licht, ed., *Therapeutic Exercise.* 2nd Ed. Baltimore: Waverly Press, 1965. P. 826.

115. Grezesiak, R. C.: Relaxation techniques in treatment of chronic pain. Arch. Phys. Med. Rehabil., *58*, June 1977.

116. Segal, J.: Biofeedback as a medical treatment. JAMA, *232* (2), Apr. 1975.

117. Knott, M.: Neuromuscular facilitation in the treatment of rheumatoid arthritis. J. Am. Phys. Ther., *44*:737, Aug. 1964.

118. Voss, D. E.: Proprioceptive neuromuscular facilitation. Am. J. Phys. Med., *46*:838, Feb. 1967.

119. Long, D. M.: Electrical stimulation for relief of pain from chronic nerve injury. J. Neurosurg., *39*:718, 1973.

120. Kabat, H.: "Chapter 13. Proprioceptive Facilitation in Therapeutic Exercise," *in* S. Licht, ed., *Therapeutic Exercise.* 2nd Ed. Baltimore: Waverly Press, 1965. P. 339.

121. Lenoch, F., Kadlcova, L.: Statistical assessment of the influence of long-term rehabilitation on hand deformities in rheumatoid arthritis. A. I. R., *7*:513, Dec. 1964.

122. Woo, S. L., Matthews, J. V., Akison, W. H., et al.: Connective tissue response to immobility. Correlative study of biomechanical and biochemical measurements of normal and immobilized rabbit knees. Arthritis Rheum., *18*:257, May–June 1975.

123. Radin, E. L., Paul, I. L.: Joint function. Arthritis Rheum., *13*:276, May–June 1970.

124. Radin, E. L., Paul, I. L., Swann, D. A., et al.: Lubrication of synovial membrane. Ann. Rheum. Dis., *30*:322, May 1971.

125. Cooke, A. F., Dowson, D., and Wright, V.: Lubrication of synovial membrane. Ann. Rheum. Dis., *35*:56–59, Feb. 1976.

126. Wright, V., Dowson, D., Longfield, M. D.: Joint stiffness — its characterization and significance. Biomed. Eng., *4*:8, Jan. 1969.

127. Baier, R. E., Shafrin, E. G., Zisman, W. A.: Adhesion: Mechanisms that assist or impede it. Science, *162*:1360, Dec. 1968.

128. Kottke, F. J., Pauley, D. L., Ptak, R. A.: The rationale for prolonged stretching for correction of shortening of connective tissue. Arch. Phys. Med., *47*:345, June 1966.

129. Van Brocklin, J. D., Ellis, D. G.: A study of the mechanical behavior of toe extensor tendons under applied stress. Arch. Phys. Med., *46*:369, May 1965.

130. Tkaczuk, H.: Tensile properties of human lumbar longitudinal ligaments. Acta Orthop. Scand. Suppl. *115*: P. 64, 1968.

131. Wright, D. G., Rennels, D. C.: A study of the elastic properties of plantar fascia. J. Bone Joint Surg., *64A*:482, Apr. 1964.

132. Swezey, R. L.: Dynamic factors in deformity of the rheumatoid arthritic hand. Bull. Rheum. Dis., *22* (1–2): 649, Series 1971–1972.

133. Swezey, R. L., Fiegenberg, D. S.: Inappropriate intrinsic muscle action in the rheumatoid hand. Ann. Rheum. Dis., *30*:619, Nov. 1971.

134. Lazarus, G. S., Brown, R. S., Daniels, J. R., et al.: Collagenolytic activity of synovium in rheumatoid arthritis. N. Engl. J. Med., *279*:914, Oct. 1968.

135. Harris, E. D., Jr., Evanson, J. M., DiBona, D. R., et al.: Collagenase and rheumatoid arthritis. Arthritis Rheum., *13*:83, Jan.–Feb. 1970.

136. Harris, E. D., Jr., Krane, S. M.: Collagenases (2nd of 3 parts). N. Engl. J. Med., *291* (12):605, 1974.

137. Nordschow, C. D.: Aspects of aging in human collagen: an exploratory thermoelastic study. Exp. Molec. Path., *5*:350, Aug. 1966.

138. Helfman, M., Bibby, B. G.: Effect of tension on lysis of collagen. Proc. Soc. Exp. Biol. Med., *126*:561, Nov. 1967.

139. Swaim, L. T.: Orthopedic and physical therapeutic treatment of chronic arthritis. JAMA, *103*:1589, Nov. 1934.

140. Agudelo, C. A., Schumacher, H. R., Phelps, P.: Effect of exercise on urate crystal–induced inflammation in canine joints. Arthritis Rheum., *15*:609, Nov.–Dec. 1972.

141. Ehrlich, G. E.: "Chapter 3. Rest and splinting," *in* G. E. Ehrlich, ed., *Total Management of the Arthritic Patient*. Philadelphia: J. B. Lippincott Co., 1973. Pp. 47 and 57.

142. Preston, R. L.: *The Surgical Management of Rheumatoid Arthritis*. Philadelphia: W. B. Saunders Co., 1968. Pp. 77, 203, 214–219, 288.

143. American Rheumatism Association, Arthritis and Rheumatism Foundation and National Institute of Arthritis and Metabolic Diseases: *Chapter 3. Evaluation of Splinting*. Criteria for and evaluation of orthopedic measures in the management of deformities of rheumatoid arthritis. Arthritis Rheum., *7*, Part 2:585, 1964.

144. Stein, H., Dickson, R. A.: Reversed dynamic slings for knee-flexion contractures in the hemophiliac. J. Bone Joint Surg., *57A*:282, Mar. 1975.

145. Reich, R. S.: "The treatment of flexion deformities of the knee as a complication of rheumatoid arthritis," *in* J. Goslings, and H. Van Swaay, eds., *Contemporary Rheumatology*. Proceedings 3rd Rheumatology Congress. New York: Elsevier Publishing Co., 1956. P. 530.

146. Williams, D.: *Functional Dynamic Slings for Knee Flexion Contractures in Chronic Rheumatic Disease*. A clinical exhibit presented at the XIV International Congress of Rheumatology, San Francisco, CA, June 26 to July 1, 1977.

147. Adamson, J. E.: Treatment of the stiff hand. Orthop. Clin. North Am., *1* (2):467, 1970.

148. Karten, I., Koatz, A. O., McEwen, C.: Treatment of contractures of the knee in rheumatoid arthritis. Bull. N. Y. Acad. Med., *44*:763, July 1968.

149. Rhinelander, F. W., Ropes, M. W.: Adjustable casts in the treatment of joint deformities. J. Bone Joint Surg., *27*:311, Apr. 1945.

150. Flatt, A. E.: "Chapter 3. Nonoperative treatment," *in* A. E. Flatt, ed., *The Care of the Rheumatoid Hand*. 3rd Ed. St. Louis: C. V. Mosby Co., 1974. P. 33.

151. Bunnell, S.: *Surgery of the Hand.* 5th Ed. Revised by J. H. Boyes. Philadelphia: J. B. Lippincott Co., 1970. P. 297.

152. Fried, D. M.: "Chapter 13. Splints for arthritis," *in* S. Licht, ed., *Arthritis and Physical Medicine.* Baltimore: Waverly Press, 1969.

153. Swezey, R. L.: Essentials of physical management and rehabilitation in arthritis. Semin. Arthritis Rheum., *3*:349, Summer 1974.

154. Kottke, F. J.: "Chapter 16. Therapeutic Exercise," *in* F. H. Krusen, F. J. Kottke, and P. M. Ellwood, eds., *Handbook of Physical Medicine and Rehabilitation.* 2nd Ed. Philadelphia: W. B. Saunders Co., 1971. Pp. 391–399.

155. Edington, D. W., Edgerton, V. R.: *The Biology of Physical Activity.* Boston: Houghton Mifflin Company, 1976. Pp. 55, 280.

156. Eysenck, H. J.: A new theory of post-rest upswing or "warm-up" in motor learning. Percept. Motor Skills, *28*:992, June 1969.

157. Kendall, P. H.: "Chapter 26. Exercise for arthritis," *in* S. Licht, ed., *Therapeutic Exercise.* 2nd Ed. New Haven: E. Licht, 1965. P. 707.

158. Cailliet, R.: *Shoulder Pain.* Philadelphia: F. A. Davis Company, 1966. P. 45.

159. Zislis, J. M.: "Chapter 12. Hydrotherapy," *in* F. H. Krusen, F. K. Kottke, and P. M. Ellwood, eds. *Handbook of Physical Medicine.* 2nd Ed. Philadelphia: W. B. Saunders Co., 1971. Pp. 346–361.

160. Hill, A. V.: Maximum work and mechanical efficiency of human muscles and their most economical speed. J. Physiol., *56*:19, Feb. 1922.

161. Osternig, L. R., Bates, B. T., James, S. L.: Isokinetic and isometric torque force relationships. Arch. Phys. Med. Rehabil., *58*:P. 254, June 1977.

162. Lehmann, J. F., et al.: Stroke: does rehabilitation affect outcome? Arch. Phys. Med. Rehabil., *56* (9):375, 1975.

163. Williams, R. B., Jr., et al.: The use of a therapeutic milieu on a continuing care unit in a general hospital. Ann. Int. Med., *73*:957, Dec. 1970.

164. Gordon, E. E., Kowalski, K., Fritts, M.: Changes in rat muscle fiber with forceful exercises. Arch. Phys. Med. Rehabil., *48*:577, Nov. 1967.

165. Hettinger, T.: Physiology of Strength. Edited by Thrulwell, M. H. Springfield, Illinois: Charles C Thomas, 1961.

166. Hines, T. F.: "Chapter 8. Manual muscle examination," *in* S. Licht, ed., *Therapeutic Exercise.* New Haven: E. Licht, 1965. Pp. 163, 175.

167. Daniels, L., Worthingham, C. A.: *Muscle Testing: Techniques of Manual Manipulation.* 3rd Ed. Philadelphia: W. B. Saunders Co., 1972. P. 16.

168. Kira, A.: Housing needs of the aged with a guide to functional planning for the elderly and handicapped. Rehabil. Lit., *21*:370, Dec. 1960.

169. Rose, D. L., Page, P. B.: Conscious proprioception and increase in muscle strength. Arch. Phys. Med., *50*:6, Jan. 1969.

170. DeLateur, B. J., Lehmann, J. F., Fordyce, W. E.: A test of the DeLorme axiom. Arch. Phys. Med. Rehabil., *49*:245, May 1968.

171. Monod, H., Sherrer, J.: Capacitée de travail statique d'un groupe musculaire synergique chez l'homme. C. R. Soc. Biol., Paris, *151*:1358, 1957.

172. Rohmert, W.: Determination of the recovery pause for static work of man. Int. Z. Angew. Physiol., *18*:123, 1960. (Ger.)

173. Müller, E. A.: Influence of training and of inactivity on muscle strength. Arch. Phys. Med., *51*:449, Aug. 1970.

174. Liberson, W. T., Asa, M. M.: Further studies of brief isometric exercises. Arch. Phys. Med. Rehabil., *40*:330, Aug. 1959.

175. Gans, B. M., Noordergraaf, A.: Voluntary skeletal muscles: a unifying theory on the relationship of their electrical and mechanical activities. Arch. Phys. Med. Rehabil., *56*:194, May 1975.

176. Milner-Brown, H. S., Stein, R. B., Lee, R. G.: Synchronization of human motor units: possible roles of exercise and supraspinal reflexes. Electroencephalogr. Clin. Neurophysiol., *38*:245, Mar. 1975.

177. Diamond, M. D., Weiss, A. J., and Grynbaum, B.: The unmotivated patient. Arch. Phys. Med., *49*:281, May 1968.

178. Hellebrandt, F. A.: Special review. Application of the overload principle to muscle training in man. Am. J. Phys. Med., *37*:278, Oct. 1958.

179. Downey, J. A., Darling, R. C., eds.: *Physiological Basis of Rehabilitation Medicine.* (Chapters 8–12) Philadelphia: W. B. Saunders Co., 1971.

180. Darling, R. C.: "Chapter 9. Exercise," *in* J. A. Downey, R. C. Darling, eds., *Physiological Basis of Rehabilitation Medicine.* Philadelphia: W. B. Saunders Co., 1971.

181. Barnard, R. J., Edgerton, V. R., Peter, J. B.: Effect of exercise on skeletal muscle. I. Biochemical and histochemical properties. J. Appl. Physiol., *28*:762, June 1970.

182. Barnard, R. J., Edgerton, V. R., Peter, J. B.: Effect of exercise on skeletal muscle. II. Contractile properties. J. Appl. Physiol., *28*:767, June 1970.

183. Jaweed, M. M., et al.: Endurance and strengthening exercise adaptations: I. Protein changes in skeletal muscles. Arch. Phys. Med. Rehabil., *55*:513, Nov. 1974.

184. Jaweed, M. M., Herbison, G. J., Gordon, E. E.: Histochemical response of rat phosphorylase to different workloads after tenotomy of the synergists. Arch. Phys. Med. Rehabil., *55*:198, May 1974.

185. Herbison, G. J., Jaweed, M. M., Ditunno, J. F.: Synergistic tenotomy: effect on chronically denervated slow and fast muscles of rats. Arch. Phys. Med. Rehabil., *56*:483, Nov. 1975.

186. George, J. C., Berger, A. J.: *Avian Myology.* New York: Academic Press, 1966. P. 77.

187. Gollnick, P. D., Armstrong, R. B., Saltin, B., et al.: Effect of training on enzyme activity and fiber composition of human skeletal muscle. J. Appl. Physiol., *34*:107, Jan. 1973.

188. Edstrom, L.: Selective changes in sizes of red and white muscle fibers in upper motor lesions and Parkinsonism. J. Neurol. Sci., *11*:537, Dec. 1970.

189. Brooke, M. H., Engel, W. K.: The histographic analysis of human muscle biopsies with regard to fiber type. 2. Diseases of the upper and lower motor neuron. Neurology, *19*:378, Apr. 1969.

190. Awad, E. A., Ibrahim, G. A., Kottke, F. J.: Structural and chemical changes in rat muscle following tenotomy. Arch. Phys. Med. Rehabil., *55* (5):193, 1974.

191. Gollnick, P. D., Armstrong, R. B., Saubert, C. W., 4th, et al.: Enzyme activity and fiber composition in skeletal muscle of untrained and trained men. J. Appl. Physiol., *33*:312, Sept. 1972.

192. Eriksson, B. O., Gollnick, P. D., and Saltin, B.: The effect of physical training on muscle enzyme activities and fiber composition in eleven-year-old boys. Acta Paediatr., Belg., *18* (Suppl.):245, 1974.

193. Gollnick, P. D., Karlsson, J., Piehl, K., et al.: Selective glycogen depletion in skeletal muscle fibers of man following sustained contractions. J. Physiol. *241*:59, Aug. 1974.

194. Müller, E. A.: Training muscle strength. Ergonomics, *2* (2):216, 1959.

195. Rose, D. L., Radzyminski, S. F., Beatty, R. R.: Effect of brief maximal exercise on the strength of the quadriceps femoris. Arch. Phys. Med. Rehabil., *38*:157, Mar. 1957.

196. Mundale, M. O.: The relationship of intermittent isometric exercise to fatigue of hand grip. Arch. Phys. Med. Rehabil., *51*:532, Sept. 1970.

197. Grimby, G., et al.: Muscle strength and endurance after training with repeated maximal isometric contractions. Scand. J. Rehabil. Med., *5* (3):118, 1973.

198. DeLorme, T. L., Watkins, A. L.: Technics of progressive resistance exercise. Arch. Phys. Med. Rehabil., *29*:263, May 1948.

199. DeLateur, B. J., Lehmann, J. F., Giaconi, R.: Mechanical work and fatigue: their roles in the development of muscle work capacity. Arch. Phys. Med. Rehabil., *57*:319, July 1976.

200. Castillo, B. A., El Sallab, R. A., Scott, J. T.: Physical activity, cystic erosions, and osteoporosis in rheumatoid arthritis. Ann. Rheum. Dis., *24*:522, Nov. 1965.

201. Jayson, M. I. V., Rubenstein, D., Dixon, A. S.: Intra-articular pressure and rheumatoid geodes (bone cysts). Ann. Rheum. Dis., *29*:496, Sept. 1970.

202. Machover, S., Sapecky, A. J.: Effect of isometric exercise on the quadriceps muscle in patients with rheumatoid arthritis. Arch. Phys. Med., *47*:737, Nov. 1966.

203. Tiselius, P.: Chapter 5. Studies on muscle weakness in rheumatoid arthritis. Acta Rheum. Scand. (Suppl.) *14*:75, 1969.

204. Jayson, M. I. V., Rubenstein, D.: Intra-articular pressure and rheumatoid geodes (bone cysts). Ann. Rheum. Dis., *29*:496, Sept. 1970.

205. Ekblom, B., Lovgren, O., Alderin, M., Fridstrom, M., Satterstrom, G. Effect of short-term physical training on patients with rheumatoid arthritis II. Scand. J. Rheum., *4* (2):87, 1975.

206. Fowler, W. M., Jr., et al.: Ineffective treatment of muscular dystrophy with an anabolic steroid and other measures. N. Engl. J. Med., *272* (17):875, 1965.

207. Vignos, P. J., Jr., Watkins, M. P.: The effect of exercise in muscular dystrophy. JAMA, *197*:843, Sept. 1966.

208. Magness, J. L., Lillegard, C., Sorensen, S., et al.: Isometric strengthening of hip muscles using a belt. Arch. Phys. Med. Rehabil., *52*:158, Apr. 1971.

209. Swezey, R. L.: Exercises with a beach ball for increasing range of joint motion. Arch. Phys. Med., *48*:253, May 1967.

210. Harris, R.: "Chapter 19. Rehabilitation," *in* S. Licht, ed., *Arthritis and Physical Medicine.* Baltimore: Waverly Press, 1969. P. 458.

211. Hellebrandt, F. A., Hautz, S. J.: Mechanism of muscle training in man: experimental demonstration of the overload principle. Phys. Ther. Rev., *36*:371, 1956.

212. Toohey, P., Larson, C. W.: *Range of Motion Exercise: Key to Joint Mobility.* Rehabilitation Publication No. 703, Sister Kenny Institute, Minneapolis, Minnesota, 1968. Pp. 2–39.

213. Bens, D. E., Krewer, S. E.: The hand gym: An exercise apparatus for the patient with rheumatoid arthritis. Arch. Phys. Med. Rehabil., *55*:477, Oct. 1974.

214. Pellegrino, E., Jr.: Physical therapy of the rheumatoid hand. Wisconsin Med. J., *66*:103, Feb. 1967.

215. Shapiro, J.: Ulnar drift: report of a related finding. Acta Orthop. Scand., *39* (3):346, 1968.

216. Pahle, J. A., Raunio, P.: The influence of wrist position on finger deviation in the rheumatoid hand. J. Bone Joint Surg., *51B*:664, Nov. 1969.

217. Bland, J. H.: *Arthritis; Medical Treatment and Home Care.* 7th Ed. New York: Collier Book, Macmillan Publishing Co., 1976. Pp. 158–168.

218. Stener, B.: Experimental evaluation of the hypothesis of ligamento-muscular protective reflexes. I. A method for adequate stimulation of tension receptors in the medial collateral ligament of the knee joint of the cat, and studies of the innervation of the ligament. Acta Physiol. Scand., *48* (Suppl. 166):5, 1959.

219. Fried, D. M.: "Chapter 12. Rest versus activity," *in* S. Licht, ed., *Arthritis and Physical Medicine.* Baltimore: Waverly Press, 1969. P. 270.

220. "Home Care Programs in Arthritis." The Arthritis Foundation, New York, 1969. Pp. 8–12.

221. Cailliet, R.: *Knee Pain and Disability.* Philadelphia: F. A. Davis Company, 1973. P. 57.

222. Cailliet, R.: *Foot and Ankle Pain.* Philadelphia: F. A. Davis Company, 1968. Pp. 89–110.

223. Duthie, R. B., Ferguson, A. B., eds.: *Mercer's Orthopaedic Surgery.* 7th Ed. Baltimore: Williams and Wilkins Co., 1973. Pp. 803–805.

224. Koepke, G. H.: "Chapter 7. Electrodiagnosis in the differential diagnosis of neck and arm pain," *in* R. W. Bailey, ed., *The Cervical Spine.* Philadelphia: Lea & Febiger, 1974. P. 115.

225. Roos, D. B., Owens, J. C.: Thoracic outlet syndrome. Arch. Surg., *93*:71, Jul. 1966.

226. Lang, E. K.: Neurovascular compression syndromes. Dis. Chest, *50*:572, Dec. 1966.

227. Britt, L. P.: Nonoperative treatment of the thoracic outlet syndrome symptoms. Clin. Orthop., *51*:45, Mar.–Apr. 1967.

228. Williams, P. C.: The conservative management of lesions of the lumbo-sacral spine. The American Academy of Orthopaedic Surgeons. Instructional Course Lectures. Michigan: American Academy of Orthopaedic Surgeons. 1953. P. 90.

229. Kendall, P. H., Jenkins, J. M.: Lumbar isometric flexion exercises. Physiotherapy, *54*:158, 1968.

230. Pearce, J., Moll, J. M.: Conservative treatment and natural history of acute lumbar disc lesions. J. Neurol. Neurosurg. Psychiat., *30*:13, Feb. 1967.

231. Nachemson, A., Lindh, M.: Measurement of abdominal and back muscle strength with and without low back pain. Scand. J. Rehabil. Med., *1* (2):60, 1969.

232. Lidstrom, A., Zachrisson, M.: Physical therapy on low back pain and sciatica. Scand. J. Rehabil. Med., *2* (1):37, 1970.

233. Nachemson, A.: Towards a better understanding of low-back pain: a review of the mechanics of the lumbar disc. Rheum. Rehabil., *14*:129, Aug. 1975.

234. Cailliet, R.: *Low Back Pain Syndrome.* 2nd Ed. Philadelphia: F. A. Davis Company, 1965. Pp. 58–70.

235. Ferderber, M. B.: Long-term illness. Management of the chronically ill patient. Penn. Med. J., *63* (3):1, 1960.
236. Cordery, J.: The conservation of physical resources as applied to the activities of patients with arthritis and the connective tissue diseases. Study Course III, Third International Congress, World Federation of Occupational Therapists. Dubuque, Iowa: William C. Brown Co., 1962. P. 22.
237. Accent on Living, Inc. Gillum Road and High Drive, P. O. Box 700, Bloomington, Illinois 61701. n.d.
238. May, E. E., Waggoner, N. R., Hotte, E. B.: *Independent Living for the Handicapped and the Elderly.* Boston: Houghton Mifflin Company, 1974. Pp. 120, 251.
239. Lowman, E. W., Klinger, J. L.: *Aids to Independent Living; Self-Help for the Handicapped.* New York: McGraw-Hill, Inc. 1969.
240. The Independence Factory. P. O. Box 597, Milltown, O. 45042. n.d.
241. *Do It Yourself Again.* The American Health Association. New York, 1965.
242. Rehabilitation Equipment and Devices Constructed in Wood. Rehabilitation Monograph XXXVI. Institute of Rehabilitation Medicine, Occupational Therapy, New York University Medical Center, 1968.
243. Brown, M. E.: "Chapter 25. Self-help clothing," *in* S. Licht, H. Kamenetz, eds., *Orthotics Etcetera.* New Haven: E. Licht, 1966. P. 601.
244. Hopkins, H. L.: "Chapter 26. Self-help aids," *in* S. Licht, H. Kamenetz, eds., *Orthotics Etcetera.* New Haven: E. Licht, 1966. P. 646.
245. Talbot, B.: "Chapter 27. Automobile modifications for disabled," *in* S. Licht, H. Kamenetz, eds., *Orthotics Etcetera.* New Haven: E. Licht, 1966. P. 676.
246. *The Functional Home for Easier Living.* Institute of Physical Medicine and Rehabilitation, New York University Medical Center, New York. n.d.
247. Hines, T. F.: "Chapter 20. Posture," *in* S. Licht, ed., *Therapeutic Exercise.* 2nd Ed. Baltimore: Waverly Press, 1965. P. 486.
248. Wheeler, R. H., Hooley, A. M.: *Physical Education for the Handicapped.* Philadelphia: Lea & Febiger, 1969.
249. Kendall, H. O., Kendall, F. P., Boynton, D. A.: *Posture and Pain.* Baltimore: Williams and Wilkins, 1952.
250. Eklundh, M.: *Spare Your Back.* London: Gerald Duckworth Co. Ltd., 1966.
251. Keegan, J. J.: Alterations of lumbar curve related to posture and seating. J. Bone Joint Surg., *35A*:589, July 1953.
252. Ellwood, P. M., Jr.: "Chapter 17. Transfers — method, equipment and preparation," *in* F. H. Krusen, F. J. Kottke, P. M. Ellwood, eds., *Handbook of Physical Medicine and Rehabilitation.* 2nd Ed. Philadelphia: W. B. Saunders Co., 1971. P. 429.
253. Davis, P. R., Troup, J. D., Burnard, J. H.: Movements of the thoracic and lumbar spine when lifting: a chrono-cyclophotographic study. J. Anat., *99*:13, Jan. 1965.
254. Preston, G. M.: Advice on housework for patients with low back pain. Occup. Ther., P. 24, Mar. 1967.
255. Nachemson, A., Elfström, G.: *Intravital Dynamic Pressure Measurements in Lumbar Discs; a Study of Common Movements, Maneuvers and Exercises.* Stockholm: Almqvist & Wiksell, 1970.
256. *Back Care.* Washington: Medic Publishing Co., n.d.
257. Knapp, M. E.: Practical physical medicine and rehabilitation. Lecture 9: Low back pain. I. Diagnosis. Postgrad. Med., *41*:A133, Feb. 1967.
258. Malick, M. H.: *Manual on Dynamic Hand Splinting with Thermoplastic Materials.* Pittsburgh, PA: Harmarville Rehabilitation Center, 1974.
259. Rizzo, F., Hamilton, B. B., Keagy, R. D.: Orthotics research evaluation framework. Arch. Phys. Med. Rehabil., *56*:304, July 1975.
260. Lusskin, R.: The influence of errors in bracing upon deformity of the lower extremity. Arch. Phys. Med. Rehabil., *47*:520, Aug. 1966.
261. Norton, P. L., Brown, T.: The immobilizing efficiency of back braces. J. Bone Joint Surg., *39A* (1):111, 1957.
262. Lumsden, R. M., Morris, J. M.: An in vivo study of axial rotation and immobilization at the lumbosacral joint. J. Bone Joint Surg., *50A*:1591, Dec. 1968.
263. Smith, E. M., Juvinall, R. C.: "Chapter 2. Mechanics of bracing," *in* S. Licht, H. Kamenetz, eds., *Orthotics Etcetera.* New Haven: E. Licht, 1966. P. 32.
264. Lehmann, J. F., Warren, C. G.: Restraining forces in various designs of knee ankle

orthoses: their placement and effect on the anatomical knee joint. Arch. Phys. Med. Rehabil., *57*:430, Sept. 1976.

265. Rotstein, J.: Use of splints in conservative management of acutely inflamed joints in rheumatoid arthritis. Arch. Phys. Med., *46*:198, Feb. 1965.

266. Rhinelander, F. W.: The effectiveness of splinting and bracing on rheumatoid arthritis. Arthritis Rheum., *2*:270, June 1959.

267. Nicholas, J. J., Ziegler, R. N.: Cylinder splints: their use in the treatment of arthritis of the knee. Arch. Phys. Med. Rehabil., *58*, June 1977.

268. Rotstein, J.: *Simple Splinting.* Philadelphia: W. B. Saunders Co., 1965.

269. Kelly, M.: The correction and prevention of deformity in rheumatoid arthritis. Active immobilization. Canad. M. A. J., *81*:827, 1959.

270. Harris, R.: "Chapter 14. Plaster splints for rheumatoid arthritis," *in* S. Licht, H. Kamenetz, eds., *Orthotics Etcetera.* New Haven: E. Licht, 1966. Pp. 336–346.

271. Faüreau, J. C., Laurin, C. A.: Joint effusions and flexion deformities. Can. M. A. J., *88*:575, Mar. 1963.

272. Jayson, M. I., Dixon, A. S.: Intra-articular pressure in rheumatoid arthritis of the knee. Pressure changes during joint use. Ann. Rheum. Dis., *29*:401, July 1970.

273. DeAndrade, J. R., Grant, C., Dixon, A. S.: Joint distension and reflex muscle inhibition in the knee. J. Bone Joint Surg., *47A*:313, Mar. 1965.

274. Ekholm, J., Eklund, G., Skoglund, S.: On the reflex effects from the knee joint of the cat. Acta Physiol. Scand., *50*:167, Oct. 1960.

275. Petersen, I., Stener, B.: Experimental evaluation of the hypothesis of ligamento-muscular protective reflexes. III. A study in man using the medial collateral ligament of the knee joint. Acta Physiol. Scand., *48* (Suppl. 166):51, 1959.

276. Andersson, S., Stener, B.: Experimental evaluation of the hypothesis of ligamento-muscular protective reflexes. Acta Physiol. Scand., *48* (Suppl. 166):33, 44–47, 1959–1960.

277. Cohen, L. A., Cohen, M. L.: Arthrokinetic reflex of the knee. Am. J. Physiol., *184*:433, Feb. 1956.

278. Palmer, I.: Pathophysiology of the medial ligament of the knee joint. Acta Chir. Scand., *115*:312, 1958.

279. Gardner, E.: Reflex muscular responses to stimulation of articular nerves in the cat. Am. J. Physiol., *161*:133, 1950.

280. Bunnell, S.: *Surgery of the Hand.* 5th Ed. Revised by Boyes, J. H. Philadelphia: J. B. Lippincott Co., 1970. Pp. 533–539.

281. Bunnell, S.: *Surgery of the Hand.* 3rd Ed. Philadelphia: J. B. Lippincott Co., 1956. Pp. 539, 552–554.

282. Marmor, L.: "Chapter 10. Surgical management of arthritis," *in* S. Licht, ed., *Arthritis and Physical Medicine.* Baltimore: Waverly Press, 1969. P. 256.

283. Millender, L. H., Nalebuff, E. A.: Arthrodesis of the rheumatoid wrist. An evaluation of 60 patients and a description of a different surgical technique. J. Bone Joint Surg., *55A*:1026, July 1973.

284. DePalma, A. F.: Diseases of the Knee. Philadelphia: J. B. Lippincott Co., 1954. P. 673.

285. Malick, M. H.: *Manual on Static Hand Splinting.* Vol. 1. Pittsburgh, PA.: Harmarville Rehabilitation Center, 1972. Pp. 32, 45, 76, 93.

286. Barr, N. R.: "Chapter 6. Choice of splinting materials," *in The Hand: Principles and Techniques of Simple Splintmaking in Rehabilitation.* Boston: Butterworth, 1975.

287. Bennett, R. L.: "Wrist and hand slip-on splints," *in* S. Licht, ed., *Arthritis and Physical Medicine.* Baltimore: Waverly Press, 1969. P. 482.

288. Granger, C. V., et al.: Laminated plaster-plastic bandage splints. Arch. Phys. Med. Rehabil., *46*:585, Aug. 1965.

289. Bennett, R. L.: Orthotic devices to prevent deformities of the hand in rheumatoid arthritis. Arthritis Rheum., *8*:1006, Oct. 1965.

290. Weatherill, F. H.: Materials for splinting; royalite, polyester resin and silastic foam in the occupational therapy clinic. Am. J. Occup. Ther., *19*:269, Sept.–Oct. 1965.

291. Morris, J. M., Lucas, D. B.: Physiological considerations in bracing of the spine. Orth. Prosthetic Appliance J., P. 37, March 1963.

292. Flatt, A. E.: "Chapter 10. Ulnar drift," *in The Care of the Rheumatoid Hand.* 3rd Ed. St. Louis: C. V. Mosby Company, 1974. P. 249.

293. Quest, I. M., Cordery, J.: A functional ulnar deviation cuff for the rheumatoid deformity. Am. J. Occup. Ther., *25*:32, Jan. 1971.

294. Ulnar Deviation Splints. Orthoplast Splint Pattern No. 2. Johnson & Johnson. (Trademark J. & J. 9027BE.)

295. Hammond, J. L.: Prevention and/or correction of ulnar deviation and pain in the rheumatoid hand. Abstract, Program 39th Annual Meeting of the American Rheumatism Association Section of the Arthritis Foundation, New Orleans, June 5, 1975. P. 114.

296. Convery, F. R., Conaty, J. P., Nickel, V. L.: Dynamic splinting of the rheumatoid hand. Orthop. Prosthet., P. 41, March 1968.

297. Van Brocklin, J. D.: Splinting the rheumatoid hand. Arch. Phys. Med., *47*:262–265, Apr. 1966.

298. Bunnell, S.: *Surgery of the Hand.* 5th Ed. Revised by Boyes, J. H. Philadelphia: J. B. Lippincott Co., 1970. Pp. 171–176.

299. Cailliet, R.: *Hand Pain and Impairment.* Philadelphia: F. A. Davis Co., 1971. P. 151.

300. Keegan, J. J.: Alterations of the lumbar curve related to posture and seating. J. Bone Joint Surg., *35A*:589, July 1953.

301. Long, C.: "Chapter 10. Upper limb bracing," *in* S. Licht, H. Kamenetz, eds., *Orthotics Etcetera.* New Haven: E. Licht, 1966. P. 152.

302. Swezey, R. L., Spiegel, T. M., Cretin, S., Clements, P.: Evaluation of a pressure gradient glove in the management of arthritic hands. Unpublished paper, 1977.

303. Ehrlich, G. E., DiPiero, A. M.: Stretch gloves: Nocturnal use to ameliorate morning stiffness in arthritic hands. Arch. Phys. Med. Rehabil., *52*:479, 1971.

304. Askari, I., Moskowitz, R. W., Ryan, C.: Stretch gloves: A study of objective and subjective effectiveness in arthritis of the hands. Arthritis Rheum., *17*:263, 1974.

305. Deaver, G. G.: "Chapter 11. Lower limb bracing." *in* S. Licht, H. Kamenetz, eds., *Orthotics Etcetera.* New Haven: E. Licht, 1966. Pp. 249, 266.

306. Lehmann, J. F., Warren, C. G., DeLateur, B. J., et al.: Biomechanical evaluation of axial loading in ischial weight-bearing braces of various designs. Arch. Phys. Med. Rehabil., *51*:331, June 1970.

307. Lehneis, H. R., Bergofsky, E., Frisina, W.: Energy expenditure with advanced lower limb orthoses and with conventional braces. Arch. Phys. Med. Rehabil., *57*:20, Jan. 1976.

308. Corcoran, P. J., Jebsen, R. H., Brengelmann, G. L., et al.: Effects of plastic and metal leg braces on speed and energy cost of hemiparetic ambulation. Arch. Phys. Med., *51*:69, Feb. 1970.

309. Siegel, I. M.: Plastic-molded knee-ankle-foot orthoses in the treatment of Duchenne muscular dystrophy. Arch. Phys. Med. Rehabil., *56*:322, July 1975.

310. Lehmann, J. F., DeLateur, B. J., Warren, C. G., et al.: Trends in lower extremity bracing. Arch. Phys. Med. Rehabil., *51*:338, June 1970.

311. Smith, E. M., Juvinall, R. C., Corell, E. B., et al.: Bracing the unstable arthritic knee. Arch. Phys. Med. Rehabil., *51*:22, Jan. 1970.

312. Hines, T. F.: "Chapter 1. Indications and principles of bracing," *in* S. Licht, H. Kamenetz, eds., *Orthotics Etcetera.* New Haven: E. Licht, 1966. P. 24.

313. Swezey, R. L.: Below-knee weight-bearing brace for the arthritic foot. Arch. Phys. Med. Rehabil., *56*:176, Apr. 1975.

314. Jebsen, R. H., Simmons, B. C., Corcoran, P. J.: Experimental plastic short leg brace. Arch. Phys. Med., *49*:108, Feb. 1968.

315. Campbell, J. W., Inman, V. T.: Treatment of plantar fasciitis and calcaneal spurs with the UC-BL shoe insert. Clin. Orthop., (103):57, 1974.

316. Zamosky, I., Licht, S.: "Chapter 18. Shoes and their modifications," *in* S. Licht, H. Kamenetz, eds. *Orthotics Etcetera.* New Haven: E. Licht, 1966. P. 402, 432.

317. Barrett, J. P., Jr.: Plantar pressure measurements. Rational shoewear in patients with rheumatoid arthritis. JAMA, *235*:1138, Mar. 1976.

318. Green, W. T., Anderson, M.: "Discrepancy in length of the lower extremities," *in American Academy of Orthopedic Surgeons,* Instructional Course Lecture. Vol. 8. Ann Arbor: J. W. Edwards, 1951. P. 294.

319. Brewerton, D. A., et al.: Pain in the neck and arm: a multicentre trial of the effects of physiotherapy. Br. Med. J., *1*:253, 1966.

320. Jacobs, B.: "Chapter 6. The arthritic spine," *in* G. E. Ehrlich, ed., *Total Management of the Arthritic Patient*. Philadelphia: J. B. Lippincott Co., 1973. P. 139.

321. Hartman, J. T., Palumbo, R., Hill, B. J.: Cineradiography of the braced normal cervical spine. A comparative study of five commonly used cervical orthoses. J. Bone Joint Surg., *59A*:332, Apr. 1977.

322. Johnson, R. M., et al.: Functional evaluation of cervical collars and braces. Abstract, American Congress of Rehabilitation Medicine, 53rd Annual Session, San Diego, November 11, 1976.

323. Fisher, S. V., et al.: Cervical orthoses effect on cervical spine motion: roentgeno-graphic and gonimetric method of study. Arch. Phys. Med. Rehabil., *58*:109, Mar. 1977.

324. Janes, J. M., Hooshmand, H.: Severe extension-flexion injuries of the cervical spine. Mayo Clin. Proc., *40*:353, May 1965.

325. Smith, P. H., Sharp, J., Kellgren, J. A.: Natural history of rheumatoid cervical subluxations. Ann. Rheum. Dis., *31*:222, May 1972.

326. Conlon, P. W., Isdale, I. C., Rose, B. S.: Rheumatoid arthritis of the cervical spine. An analysis of 333 cases. Ann. Rheum. Dis., *25*:120, Mar. 1966.

327. Bland, J. H.: Rheumatoid arthritis of the cervical spine. Bull. Rheum. Dis., *18* (2):471, 1967.

328. Honet, J. C., Puri, K.: Cervical radiculitis: Treatment and results in 82 patients. Arch. Phys. Med. Rehabil., *57*:12, Jan. 1976.

329. Cervical-spine involvement in rheumatoid arthritis. The Lancet, *1*:586, 1973.

330. Thistle, H. G.: Neck and shoulder pain: evaluation and conservative management. Med. Clin. N. Amer., *53*:511, May 1969.

331. Redford, J. B.: "Chapter 23. Beds and Tables," *in* S. Licht, H. Kamenetz, eds., *Orthotics Etcetera*. New Haven: E. Licht, 1966. P. 566.

332. The Jackson Cervipillo Tru-Eze Mfg. Co., Inc. P.O. Box 855, Burbank, California.

333. Lucas, D. B.: "Chapter 12. Spinal bracing," *in* S. Licht, H. Kamenetz, eds., *Orthotics Etcetera*. New Haven: E. Licht, 1966, P. 291.

334. Waters, R. L., Morris, J. M.: Effect of spinal supports on the electrical activity of muscles of the trunk. J. Bone Joint Surg. (Amer.), *52*:51, Jan. 1970.

335. Perry, J.: The use of external support in the treatment of low-back pain. J. Bone Joint Surg. (Amer.), *52*:1440, 1970.

336. Morris, J. M., Lucas, D. B., Bresler, B.: Role of the trunk in stability of the spine. J. Bone Joint Surg. (Amer.), *43*:327, Apr. 1961.

337. Stillwell, G. K.: The law of Laplace. Some clinical applications. Mayo Clin. Proc., *48*:863, 1973.

338. Russek, A. S.: Biochemical and physiological basis for ambulatory treatment of low back pain. Orth. Review, *5*:21, 1976.

339. Blount, W. P.: "Chapter 13. Bracing for Scoliosis," *in* S. Licht, H. L. Kamenetz, eds. *Orthotics Etcetera*. New Haven: E. Licht, 1966. P. 306.

340. *Rehabilitative Nursing Techniques — 1: Bed Positioning and Transfer Procedures for the Hemiplegic*. Minneapolis, Minn.: Kenny Rehabilitation Institute, 1964.

341. Laging, B.: Furniture design for the elderly. Rehab. Lit., *27*:130, May 1966.

342. Travell, J.: *Ladies and Gentlemen, Be Seated — Properly*. House Beautiful, July 1961. P. 159.

343. Stoner, E. K.: "Chapter 3. Evaluation of the amputee," *in* F. H. Krusen, F. J. Kottke, P. M. Ellwood, eds., *Handbook of Physical Medicine and Rehabilitation*. 2nd Ed. Philadelphia: W. B. Saunders Co., 1971. P. 92.

344. Frankel, V. H., Burstein, A. H.: *Orthopaedic Biomechanics*. Philadelphia: Lea & Febiger, 1970. P. 35.

345. Corcoran, P. J.: "Chapter 10. Energy expenditure during ambulation," *in* J. A. Downey, R. C. Darling, eds., *Physiological Basis of Rehabilitation Medicine*. Philadelphia: W. B. Saunders Co., 1971. P. 185.

346. Dacso, M. M., Luczak, A. K., Haas, A., et al.: Bracing and rehabilitation training. Effect on the energy expenditure of the elderly hemiplegic; preliminary report. Postgrad. Med., *34*:42, July 1963.

347. Reinstein, L., Staas, W. E., Marquette, C. H.: A rehabilitation evaluation system which complements the problem-oriented medical record. Arch. Phys. Med. Rehabil., *56*:396, Sep. 1975.

348. Blount, W. P.: Don't throw away the cane. J. Bone Joint Surg., *38A*:695, 1958.

349. Sorenson, L., Ulrich, P. G.: *Ambulation: A Manual for Nurses.* Minneapolis, Minnesota: American Rehabilitation Foundation, 1966.

350. Cicenia, E. F., Hoberman, M.: Crutch management drills. Modern Medicine, *26* (9):86, 1958.

351. Kamenetz, H. L.: "Chapter 21. Wheelchairs," *in* S. Licht, H. L. Kamenetz, eds., *Orthotics Etcetera.* New Haven: E. Licht, 1966. P. 473.

352. "Wheelchair." Accent on Information Search Request Form: Bloomington, Illinois, 61701.

353. Bergstrom, D. A.: Report on a conference for wheelchair manufacturers. Bulletin of Prosthetics Research, *BPR 10–3,* Spring, 1965. P. 60.

354. Lee, M. H. M., Pezenik, D. P., Dacso, M. M.: Wheelchair prescription. Public Health Service Rehabilitation Guide, Series 1, U.S. Department of HEW. Public Health Service, Publication 1666. 1967.

355. American Automobile Association: *Vehicle Controls for Disabled Persons.* Washington, D.C., 1973.

356. The Gazette: *Vans, busses, hydraulic lifts, and public transportation.* St. Louis, Missouri: Rehabilitation Gazette, 1973.

357. "Survey of special laws for handicapped drivers." Accent on Living Magazine, Fall, 1973.

358. "Driver Education for the Handicapped." Des Moines Public School District and Younker Memorial Rehabilitation Center in cooperation with the National Highway Traffic Safety Administration and the Department of Public Instruction. n.d.

359. DeGravelles, W. D., Jr.: Evaluation of the handicapped driver. Presented at San Diego, Calif.: American Academy of Physical Medicine and Rehabilitation, June 1976.

360. Stock, M. S., Light, W. O., Douglass, J. M., et al.: Licensing the driver with musculo-skeletal difficulty. J. Bone Joint Surg. (Amer.), *52*:343, Mar. 1970.

361. Kira, A.: Housing needs of the aged with a guide to functional planning for the elderly and handicapped. Rehab. Lit., *21*:370, Dec. 1960.

362. Ramsey, C. G., Sleeper, H. R.: *Architectural Graphic Standards.* 6th Ed. New York: John Wiley & Sons, Inc., 1970. Pp. 4–5.

363. Licht, S.: "History of therapeutic heat," *in* S. Licht, ed., *Therapeutic Heat and Cold.* 2nd Ed. New Haven: E. Licht, 1965.

364. Kantor, T. G., Sunshine, A., Laska, E., et al.: Oral analgesic studies: pentazocine hydrochloride, codeine, aspirin, and placebo and their influence on response to placebo. Clin. Pharmacol. Ther., *7*:447, July–Aug. 1966.

365. Nuki, G., Downie, W. W., Dick, W. C., et al.: Clinical trials of pentazocine in rheumatoid arthritis. Observations on the value of potent analgesics and placebos. Ann. Rheum. Dis., *32*:436, Sept. 1973.

366. Famaey, J., Lee, P.: More recent non-steroidal anti-rheumatic drugs. Parts 1 and 2. Clin. Rheum. Dis., *1*:285, Aug. 1975.

367. Morison, R. A., Woodmansey, A., Young, A. J.: Placebo responses in an arthritis trial. Ann. Rheum. Dis., *20*:179, June 1961.

368. Fearnley, G. R., Lackner, R., Meanock, R. I., et al.: Pilot study of intra-articular procaine and hydrocortisone acetate in rheumatoid arthritis. Ann. Rheum. Dis., *15*:134, June 1956.

369. Mouertel, C. G., et al.: Who responds to sugar pills? Mayo Clin. Proc., *51*:96, 1976.

370. Wright, V., Hopkins, R.: Administration of antirheumatic drugs. Ann. Rheum. Dis., *35*:174, Apr. 1976.

371. O'Brien, W. M.: Indomethacin: a survey of clinical trials. Clin. Pharmacol. Ther., *9*:94, Jan.–Feb. 1968.

372. Lesse, S.: *Anxiety: Its Components, Development, and Treatment.* Chapter 10. New York: Grune and Stratton, 1970. Pp. 113–133.

373. Greene, C. S., Laskin, D. M.: Splint therapy for the myofascial pain — dysfunction (MPD) syndrome: a comparative study. J. Am. Dent. Assoc., *84*:624, Mar. 1972.

374. Schwitzgebel, R. K., Traugott, M.: Initial note on the placebo effect of machines. Behav. Sci., *13*:267, July 1968.

375. Beecher, H. K.: "Chapter 2. Placebo effects of situations, attitudes, and drugs: A quantitative study of suggestibility," *in* K. Rickels, ed., *Non-specific Factors in Drug Therapy*. Springfield: Charles C Thomas, 1968. P. 27.

376. Stillwell, G. K.: "Chapter 10. Therapeutic Heat and Cold," *in* F. H. Krusen, F. J. Kottke, P. M. Ellwood, eds., *Handbook of Physical Medicine and Rehabilitation*. 2nd Ed. Philadelphia: W. B. Saunders Co., 1971. Pp. 259–272.

377. Wells, H. S.: Temperature equalization for the relief of pain; experimental study of relation of thermal gradients to pain. Arch. Phys. Med., *28*:135, Mar. 1947.

378. Lehmann, J. F., Brunner, G. D., Stow, R. W.: Pain threshold measurement after therapeutic application of ultrasound, microwaves and infrared. Arch. Phys. Med. Rehabil., *39*:560, Sep. 1958.

379. Stuhlfauth, K.: Neural effects of ultrasonic waves. Brit. J. Phys. Med., *15*:10, Jan. 1952.

380. McAfee, R. D.: Physiological effects of thermode and microwave stimulation of peripheral nerves. Am. J. Physiol., *203*:374, Aug. 1962.

381. Hollander, J. L., Horvath, S. M.: The influence of physical therapy procedures on the intra-articular temperature of normal and arthritic subjects. Am. J. Sc. M., *218*:543, Nov. 1949.

382. Stoner, E. K.: "Chapter 9. Luminous and Infrared Heating," *in* S. Licht, ed., *Therapeutic Heat*. New Haven: E. Licht, 1958. P. 235.

383. Abramson, D. I., et al.: Comparison of wet and dry heat in raising temperature of tissues. Arch. Phys. Med. Rehabil., *48*:654, 1967.

384. Downey, J. A.: Physiological effects of heat and cold. J. Amer. Phys. Ther. Ass., *44*:713, Aug. 1964.

385. Harris, R.: The effect of various forms of physical therapy on radio-sodium clearance from the normal and arthritic knee joint. Ann. Phys. Med., 7:1, Feb. 1963.

386. Davis, F. A.: The hot bath test in the diagnosis of multiple sclerosis. J. Mount Sinai Hosp. N. Y., *33*:280, May–June 1966.

387. Millard, J. B.: "Chapter 8. Conductive Heating," *in* S. Licht, ed., *Therapeutic Heat*, New Haven: E. Licht, 1958.

388. Andrews, G. R., Ofner, F.: The limitations of reflex heating therapy in the elderly. J. Am. Geriatr. Soc., *20*:84, Feb. 1972.

389. Harris, R.: "Chapter 17. Heat in vascular disorders," *in* S. Licht, ed., *Therapeutic Heat*. New Haven: E. Licht, 1958. P. 353.

390. Knutsson, E., Martensson, E.: Effects of local cooling on monosynaptic reflexes in man. Scand. J. Rehab. Med., *1*:126, 1969.

391. Darling, R. C.: "Chapter 9. Exercise," *in* J. A. Downey, R. C. Darling, eds., *Physiological Basis of Rehabilitation Medicine*. Philadelphia: W. B. Saunders Co., 1971.

392. Benson, T. B., Copp, E. P.: The effects of therapeutic forms of heat and ice on the pain threshold of the normal shoulder. Rheum. Rehabil., *13*:101, May, 1974.

393. Dorwart, B. B., Hansell, J. R., Schumacher, H. R., Jr.: Effects of cold and heat on urate crystal–induced synovitis in the dog. Arthritis Rheum., *17*:563, 1974.

394. Olson, J. E., Stravino, V. D.: A review of cryotherapy. Phys. Ther., *52*:840, Aug. 1972.

395. Kirk, J. A., Kersley, G. D.: Heat and cold in the physical treatment of rheumatoid arthritis of the knee. A controlled clinical trial. Ann. Phys. Med., *9*:270, Aug. 1968.

396. Clarke, G. R., et al.: Evaluation of physiotherapy in the treatment of osteoarthrosis of the knee. Rheum. Rehabil., *13*:190, Nov. 1974.

397. Stimson, C. W., Rose, G. B., and Nelson, P. A.: Paraffin bath as a thermotherapy: an evaluation. Arch. Phys. Med. Rehabil., *39*:219, Apr. 1958.

398. Cordray, Y. M., Krusen, E. M.: Use of hydrocollator packs in the treatment of neck and shoulder pains. Arch. Phys. Med. Rehabil., *40*:105, Mar. 1959.

399. Harris, R., Millard, J. B.: Paraffin-wax baths in the treatment of rheumatoid arthritis. Ann. Rheum. Dis., *14*:278, Sep. 1955.

400. Landen, B. R.: Heat or cold for the relief of low back pain? Phys. Ther., *47*:1126, Dec. 1967.

401. Hansen, T. I., Kristensen, J. H.: Effect of massage, short wave diathermy and ultrasound upon ^{133}Xe disappearance rate from muscle and subcutaneous tissue of the human calf. Scand. J. Rehabil. Med., *5* (4):179, 1973.

402. Gucker, T.: "Heat and cold in orthopedics," *in* S. Licht, ed., *Therapeutic Heat and Cold.* New Haven: E. Licht, 1965. Pp. 398–406.
403. Grant, A. E.: Massage with ice (cryokinetics) in the treatment of painful conditions of the musculoskeletal system. Arch. Phys. Med., *45*:233, May 1964.
404. Matsen, F. A., Questad, K., Matsen, A. L.: The effect of local cooling on postfracture swelling: a controlled study. Clin. Orthop., *109*:201, 1975.
405. Basmajian, J. V.: Control and training of individual motor units. Science, *141*:440, Aug. 1963.
406. Schwan, H. P., Piersol, G. M.: The absorption of electromagnetic energy in body tissues; review and critical analysis; physiological and clinical aspects. Am. J. Phys. Med., *34*:425, June 1955.
407. Lehmann, J. F., McMillan, J. A., Brunner, G. D., et al.: Comparative study of the efficiency of short-wave, microwave and ultrasonic diathermy in heating the hip joint. Arch. Phys. Med. Rehabil., *40*:510, Dec. 1959.
408. Lehmann, J. F., Fordyce, W. E., Rathbun, L. A., et al.: Clinical evaluation of a new approach in the treatment of contracture associated with hip fracture after internal fixation. Arch. Phys. Med., *42*:95, Feb. 1961.
409. Lehmann, J. F., DeLateur, B. J., Warren, C. G., et al.: Heating of joint structures by ultrasound. Arch. Phys. Med., *49*:28, Jan. 1968.
410. Hovind, H., Nielsen, S. L.: Local blood flow after short-wave diathermy. Preliminary report. Arch. Phys. Med. Rehabil., *55*:217, May 1974.
411. Bach, S. A., Luzzio, A. J., Brownell, A. S.: "Effects of radio-frequency energy on human gamma globulin," *in* M. E. Peyton, ed., Proceedings of the 4th Annual Tri-Service Conference on the Biological Effects of Microwave Radiation, *1*:117, 1960.
412. Kottke, F. J., Koza, D. W., Kubicek, W. G., et al.: Studies of deep circulatory response to short wave diathermy and microwave diathermy in man. Arch. Phys. Med., *30*:431, Jul. 1949.
413. Lehmann, J. F., Warren, C. G., Scham, S. M.: Therapeutic heat and cold. Clin. Orthop. Related Research, *99*:207, Mar.–Apr. 1974.
414. Warren, C. G., Lehmann, J. F., Koblanski, J. N.: Heat and stretch procedures: an evaluation using rat tail tendon. Arch. Phys. Med. Rehabil., *57*:122, 1976.
415. Gersten, J. W.: Effect of ultrasound on tendon extensibility. Am. J. Phys. Med., *34*:362, 1955.
416. Lehmann, J. F., Masock, A. J., Warren, C. G., et al.: Effect of therapeutic temperatures on tendon extensibility. Arch. Phys. Med., *51*:481, Aug. 1970.
417. Fountain, F. P., Gersten, J. W., Sengir, O.: Decrease in muscle spasm produced by ultrasound, hot packs, and infrared radiation. Arch. Phys. Med., *41*:293, July 1960.
418. Soren, A.: Evaluation of ultrasound treatment in musculo-skeletal disorders. Physiotherapy, *51*:214, July 1965.
419. Lehmann, J. F.: Chapter 11. Diathermy," *in* S. Licht, ed., *Therapeutic Heat.* Baltimore: Waverly Press, Inc., 1958.
420. Lehmann, J. F., Krusen, F. H.: Biophysical effects of ultrasonic energy on carcinoma and their possible significance. Arch. Phys. Med., *36*:452, July 1955.
421. Scott, B. O.: The effects of metal on short-wave field distribution. Ann. Phys. Med., *1*:238, July 1953.
422. Feucht, B. L., Richardson, A. W., Hines, H. M.: Effects of implanted metals on tissue hyperthermia produced by microwaves. Arch. Phys. Med., *30*:164, Mar. 1949.
423. Rae, J. W., Jr., Martin, G. M., Treanor, W. J., et al.: Clinical experiences with microwave diathermy. Proc. Staff Meet. Mayo Clin., *25*:441, July 1950.
424. Addington, C. H., et al.: Biological effects of microwave energy at 200 mc. Proceedings of the 4th Annual Tri-Service Conference on the Biological Effects of Microwave Radiation, *1*:177, 1961.
425. Tomberg, V. T.: Special thermal effects of high frequency fields. Proceedings of 4th Annual Tri-Service Conference on the Biological Effects of Microwave Radiation, *1*:221, 1961.
426. Ferris, B. G., Jr.: Environmental hazards. Electromagnetic radiation. N. Engl. J. Med., *275*:1100, Nov. 1966.
427. Merckel, C.: Microwave and man. The direct and indirect hazards, and the precautions. Calif. Med., *117*:20, July 1972.

428. Overgaard, K., Overgaard, J.: Investigation on the possibility of thermic tumor therapy: I. Short-wave treatment of a transplanted isologous mammary carcinoma. Eur. J. Cancer, *8*:65, 1972.

429. Hahn, G. M., Boone, M. L. M.: Heat in tumor therapy. (Letter.) J.A.M.A., *236*:2286, Nov. 1976.

430. Doss, J. D., McCabe, C. W.: A technique for localized heating in tissue: An adjunct to tumor therapy. Med. Instrum., *10*:16, Jan.–Feb. 1976.

431. Scott, B. O.: "Short Wave Diathermy," *in* S. Licht, ed., *Therapeutic Heat and Cold.* 2nd Ed. New Haven: E. Licht, 1965. Pp. 275–309.

432. Lehmann, J. F.: New microwave applicators and their evaluation with specific reference to the new standards. Read at the Northwest Association of Physical Medicine and Rehabilitation, Annual Meeting, Portland, Oregon, April, 1976.

433. Lehmann, J. F.: "Chapter 11. Diathermy," *in* F. H. Krusen, F. J. Kottke, P. M. Ellwood, eds., *Handbook of Physical Medicine and Rehabilitation.* 2nd Ed. Philadelphia: W. B. Saunders Co., 1971. Pp. 273–345.

434. Lehmann, J. F., Brunner, G. D., Martinez, A. J., et al.: Ultrasonic effects as demonstrated in live pigs with surgical metallic implants. Arch. Phys. Med. Rehabil., *40*:483, Nov. 1959.

435. Lehmann, J. F., et al.: Comparison of ultrasonic and microwave diathermy in the physical treatment of periarthritis of the shoulder. (Study of the effects of ultrasonic and microwave diathermy when employed in conjunction with massage and exercise). Arch. Phys. Med., *35*:627, Oct. 1954.

436. Harris, E. D., Jr., McCroskery, P. A.: The influence of temperature and fibril stability on degradation of cartilage collagen by rheumatoid synovial collagenase. N. Engl. J. Med., *290*:1, Jan. 1974.

437. Hollander, J. L.: Editorial: Collagenase, cartilage and cortisol. N. Engl. J. Med., *290*:50, Jan. 1974.

438. Feibel, A., Fast, A.: Deep heating of joints: A reconsideration. Arch. Phys. Med. Rehabil., *57*:513, 1976.

439. Lehmann, J. F., DeLateur, B. J.: "Chapter 14. Heat and Cold in the Treatment of Arthritis," *in* S. Licht, ed., *Arthritis and Physical Medicine.* New Haven: E. Licht, 1969. Pp. 315–378.

440. Harris, R.: "Chapter 8. Therapeutic pools," *in* S. Licht, ed., *Medical Hydrology.* New Haven: E. Licht, 1963. P. 189.

441. Behrend, H. J.: "Chapter 12. Hydrotherapy," *in* S. Licht, ed., *Medical Hydrology.* New Haven: E. Licht, 1963. P. 239.

442. Wilson, I. H., Kasch, S. W.: "Chapter 11. Medical Aspects of Swimming," *in* S. Licht, ed., *Medical Hydrology.* New Haven: E. Licht, 1969. P. 229.

443. Harris, R., McInnes, M.: "Chapter 9. Exercises in Water," *in* S. Licht, ed., *Medical Hydrology.* New Haven: E. Licht, 1963. P. 207.

444. Farfan, H. F.: *Mechanical Disorders of the Low Back.* Philadelphia: Lea & Febiger, 1973. Pp. 220–221.

445. Harris, R.: "Chapter 12. Traction," *in* S. Licht, ed., *Massage, Manipulation and Traction.* New Haven: E. Licht, 1960. P. 223.

446. Judovich, B. D.: Lumbar traction therapy and dissipated force factors. Lancet, *74*:411, Oct. 1954.

447. Judovich, B. D., Nobel, G. R.: Traction therapy, a study of resistance forces. Am. J. Surg., *93*:108, Jan. 1957.

448. Hood, L. B., Chrisman, D.: Intermittent pelvic traction in the treatment of the ruptured intervertebral disk. Phys. Ther., *48*:21, Jan. 1968.

449. Mathews, J. A.: Dynamic discography: a study of lumbar traction. Ann. Phys. Med., *9*:275, Aug. 1968.

450. Neuwirth, E., Hilde, W., Campbell, R.: Tables for vertebral elongation in the treatment of sciatica. Arch. Phys. Med., *33*:455, Aug. 1952.

451. Neuwirth, E.: Current status of spinal traction. Lancet, *77*:243, 1957.

452. Worden, R. E., Humphrey, T. L.: Effect of spinal traction on the length of the body. Arch. Phys. Med. Rehabil., *45*:318, 1964.

453. Lehmann, J. F., Brunner, G. D.: A device for the application of heavy lumbar traction: its mechanical effects. Arch. Phys. Med. Rehabil., *39*:696, Nov. 1958.

454. Chrisman, O. D., Mittnacht, A., Snook, G. A.: A study of the results following rotary manipulation in the lumbar intervertebral-disc syndrome. J. Bone Joint Surg. (Amer.), *46*:517, Apr. 1964.

455. Lawson, G. A., Godfrey, C. M.: A report on studies of spinal traction. Med. Serv. J. Canada, *14*:762, 1958.

456. Masturzo, A.: Vertebral traction for treatment of sciatica. Rheumatism, *11*:62, July 1955.

457. Cyriax, J.: Discussion on the treatment of backache by traction. Proc. R. Soc. Med., *48*:808, 1955.

458. Young, R. H.: "Chapter 14. The Spine — Low Back," in G. C. Lloyd-Roberts, ed., *Orthopaedics (Clinical Surgery — 13)*. London: Butterworths, 1967. P. 345.

459. Crisp, E. J.: Discussion on the treatment of backache by traction. Proc. R. Soc. Med., *48*:805, 1955.

460. Krusen, E. M.: Acute injuries to the neck. Mod. Med., *28*:200, 1960.

461. Jackson, R.: *Cervical Syndrome.* 3rd Ed. Springfield, Ill.: Charles C Thomas, 1966. Pp. 245–259.

462. Valtonen, E. J., Moller, K., Wiljasalo, M.: Comparative radiographic study of the effect of intermittent and continuous traction on elongation of the cervical spine. Ann. Med. Int. Fenn., *57*:143, 1968. (Finland)

463. Judovich, B. D.: Herniated cervical disc; new form of traction therapy. Am. J. Surg., *84*:646, Dec. 1952.

464. Williams, M., Lissner, H.: *Biomechanics of Human Motion.* Philadelphia: W. B. Saunders Co., 1962. Pp. 118–121.

465. Martin, G. M., Corbin, K. B.: An evaluation of conservative treatment for patients with cervical disk syndrome. Proc. Staff Meet. Mayo Clin., *29*:324, June 1954.

466. Martin, G. M., Corbin, K. B.: An evaluation of conservative treatment for patients with cervical disk syndrome. Arch. Phys. Med. Rehabil., *35*:87, Feb. 1954.

467. "Neckache and Backache." Proceedings of a workshop sponsored by the American Association of Neurological Surgeons in cooperation with the National Institutes of Health, Bethesda, Maryland. E. S. Gurdjian, L. M. Thomas, eds. Springfield, Ill.: Charles C Thomas, 1970.

468. Crue, B. J.: Importance of flexion in cervical traction for radiculitis. U. S. Armed Forces Med. J., *8*:378, 1957.

469. Bland, J. H.: *Arthritis: Medical Treatment and Home Care.* New York: Macmillan Co., 1960. Pp. 128–129.

470. Colachis, S. C., Jr., Strohm, B. R.: A study of tractive forces and angle of pull on vertebral interspaces in the cervical spine. Arch. Phys. Med., *46*:820, Dec. 1965.

471. Smith, B. H.: *Cervical Spondylosis and its Neurological Complications.* Springfield, Ill.: Charles C Thomas, 1968. Pp. 35–37.

472. Cailliet, R.: *Neck and Arm Pain.* Philadelphia: F. A. Davis Company, 1964. Pp. 79–82.

473. Smith, R. A., Estridge, M. N.: Neurologic complications of head and neck manipulations. JAMA, *182*:528, Nov. 1962.

474. Gurdjian, E. S., Thomas, L. M.: Neckache and Backache. A Workshop sponsored by the American Assoc. of Neurol. Surgeons in cooperation with the NIH, Bethesda, Maryland, Springfield, Ill.: Charles C Thomas, 1970.

475. Brain, L., Wilkinson, M.: *Cervical Spondylosis and Other Disorders of the Cervical Spine.* 1st Ed., London: Heineman, 1971. P. 203.

476. Licht, S.: *Massage, Manipulation and Traction.* New Haven: E. Licht, 1960. P. 104.

477. Firman, G. J., Goldstein, M. S.: The future of chiropractic: a psychosocial view. N. Engl. J. Med., *293*:639, Sep. 1975.

478. Wilbur, R. S.: What the health-care consumer should know about chiropractic. JAMA, *215*:1307, Feb. 1971.

479. American Federation of Labor and Congress of Industrial Organizations: AFL-CIO fact sheet on chiropractic. JAMA, *214*:1095, Nov. 1970.

480. Hewitt, D., Wood, P. H.: Heterodox practitioners and the availability of specialist advice. Rheum. Rehabil., *14*:191, Aug. 1975.

481. Pribek, R. A.: Brain stem vascular accident following neck manipulation. Wisconsin Med. J., *62*:141, Mar. 1963.

482. Miller, R. G., Burton, R.: Stroke following chiropractic manipulation of the spine. JAMA, *229*:189, July 1974.

483. Livingstone, M. C. P.: Spinal manipulation in medical practice: a century of ignorance. Med. J. Aust., *2*:552, Sept. 1968.

484. Maitland, G. D.: Lumbar manipulation: does it do harm? A five-year follow-up survey. Med. J. Aust., 48:546, Sept. 1961.

485. Travell, J., Travell, W.: Therapy of low back pain by manipulation and of referred pain in the lower extremity by procaine infiltration. Arch. Phys. Med., 27:537, Sept. 1946.

486. Doran, D. M., Newell, D. J.: Manipulation in treatment of low back pain: a multicentre study. Br. Med. J., 2(5964):161, Apr. 1975.

487. Cyriax, J.: Conservative treatment of lumbar disc lesions. Physiotherapy, 50:300, Sept. 1964.

488. Robertson, A. M.: The challenge of the painful back — an industrial and medical problem. Trans. Soc. Occup. Med., 20:42, Apr. 1970.

489. Glover, J. R., Morris, J. G., Khosla, T.: Back pain: a randomized clinical trial of rotational manipulation of the trunk. Br. J. In. Med., 31:59, Jan. 1974.

490. Maigne, R.: Orthopedic Medicine; a New Approach to Vertebral Manipulation. Springfield, Ill.: Charles C Thomas, 1972.

491. Cyriax, J.: "Treatment by manipulation and massage," in Textbook of Orthopaedic Medicine, Volume I. 6th Ed. Baltimore: Williams and Wilkins Co., 1975. Pp. 440–467, 699–719.

492. Mennell, J. M.: Back Pain; Diagnosis and Treatment Using Manipulative Techniques. Boston: Little, Brown Co., 1960.

493. Unsworth, A., Dowson, D., Wright, V.: Cracking joints. A bioengineering study of cavitation in the metacarpophalangeal joint. Ann. Rheum. Dis., 30:348, July 1971.

494. Mennell, J. M.: Joint Pain; Diagnosis and Treatment Using Manipulative Techniques. Boston: Little, Brown Co., 1964.

495. Kellgren, J. H.: On the distribution of pain arising from deep somatic structures with charts of segmental pain areas. Clin. Sci., 4:35, June 1939.

496. Feinstein, B., Langton, J. N. K., Jameson, R. M., et al.: Experiments on pain referred from deep somatic tissues. J. Bone Joint Surg., 36A:981, Oct. 1954.

497. Wolff, B. B., Jarvik, M. E.: Variations in cutaneous and deep somatic pain sensitivity. Canad. J. Psychol., 17:37, Mar. 1963.

498. Travell, J.: Symposium on mechanism and management of pain syndromes. Proceedings of the Rudolf Virchow Medical Society, New York, 16:1, 1957.

499. Mennell, J. M.: "Spray-and-stretch" treatment for myofascial pain. Hospital Physician, 12:47, 1973.

500. Travell, J., Rinzler, S. H.: Scientific exhibit: the myofascial genesis of pain. Postgrad. Med., 11:425, May 1952.

501. Travell, J.: Ethyl chloride spray for painful muscle spasm. Arch. Phys. Med., 33:291, May 1952.

502. Bonica, J. J.: Management of myofascial pain syndromes in general practice. JAMA, 164:732, 1957.

503. Woodbury, J. W., Ruch, T. C.: "Chapter 4. Muscle," in T. C. Ruch, J. F. Fulton, eds., Medical Physiology and Biophysics. 18th ed. of Howell's Textbook of Physiology. Philadelphia: W. B. Saunders, 1960. P. 126.

504. Norris, F. H., Gasteiger, E. L., Chatfield, P. O.: An electromyographic study of induced and spontaneous muscle cramps. EEG Clin. Neurophysiol., 9:139, 1957.

505. Attali, P., Liëvre, J. A.: Muscle contracture in low back pain and ischialgia. (Recherche de la contracture musculaire chez les sujets atteints de lombalgie et de sciatique). Rev. Rhum., 32:514, Aug.–Sep. 1965. (Fr.)

506. Arroyo, P., Jr.: Electromyography in the evaluation of reflex muscle spasm. Simplified method for direct evaluation of muscle-relaxant drugs. J. Florida Med. Ass., 53:29, Jan. 1966.

507. Cobb, C. R., deVries, H. A., Urban, R. T., et al.: Electrical activity in muscle pain. Am. J. Phys. Med., 54:80, Apr. 1975.

508. Gammon, G. D., Starr, I.: Studies on the relief of pain by counter-irritation. J. Clin. Investigation, 20:13, Jan. 1941.

509. Brown, B. R.: Office management of common musculoskeletal pain syndromes. Amer. Fam. Physician, 6:92, 1972.

510. Gorrell, R. L.: Treatment of skeletal pain with procaine injections; an analysis of 295 cases in general practice. Am. J. Surg., 63:102, Jan. 1944.

511. Dittrich, R. J.: Local anesthesia in diagnosis and treatment of low back pain. Am. Pract. & Digest. Treat., *6*:859, June 1955.

512. Pace, J. B., Nagle, D.: Piriform syndrome. West. J. Med., *124*:435, June 1976.

513. Wall, P. D., Cronly-Dillon, J. R.: Pain, itch, and vibration. AMA Arch. Neurol., *2*:365, Apr. 1960.

514. Melzack, R., Wall, P. D.: Pain mechanisms: a new theory. Science, *150*:971, Nov. 1965.

515. Campbell, J. N., Taub, A.: Local analgesia from percutaneous electrical stimulation. A peripheral mechanism. Arch. Neurol., *28*:347, May 1973.

516. Kerr, F. W. L.: Pain. A central inhibitory balance theory. Mayo Clin. Proc., *50*:685, Dec. 1975.

517. "Pain Symposium." Congress of Neurological Surgeons. Surg. Neurol., *4*:61, July 1975.

518. Sweet, W. H.: Lessons on pain control from electrical stimulation. College Physician, *35*:171, 1968.

519. Long, D. M.: External electrical stimulation as a treatment of chronic pain. Minn. Med., *57*:195, Mar. 1974.

520. Indeck, W., Printy, A.: Skin application of electrical impulses for relief of pain. Minn. Med., *58*:305, Apr. 1975.

521. Loeser, J. D., Black, R. G., Christman, A.: Relief of pain by transcutaneous stimulation. J. Neurosurg., *42*:308, Mar. 1975.

522. Shealy, C. N., Maurer, D.: Transcutaneous nerve stimulation for control of pain. A preliminary technical note. Surg. Neurol., *2*:45, Jan. 1974.

523. Ebersold, M. J., Lows, E. R., Stonnington, H. H., et al.: Transcutaneous electrical stimulation for treatment of chronic pain: a preliminary report. Surg. Neurol., *4*:96, July 1975.

524. Picaza, J. A., Cannon, B. W., Hunter, S. E., et al.: Pain suppression by peripheral nerve stimulation. Part 1. Observations with transcutaneous stimuli. Surg. Neurol., *4*:105, July 1975.

525. Thorsteinsson, G., et al.: Transcutaneous electrical stimulation: a double-blind trial of its efficacy for pain. Arch. Phys. Med. Rehabil., *58*:8, 1977.

526. Hart, F. D., Huskisson, E. C.: Pain patterns in the rheumatic disorders. Br. Med. J., *4*:213, Oct. 1972.

527. Fordyce, W. E.: An operant conditioning method for managing chronic pain. Postgrad. Med., *53*:123, Mar. 1973.

528. Swanson, D. W., Swenson, W. M., Morida, T.: Program for managing chronic pain. 1. Program description and characteristics of patients. Mayo Clin. Proc., *51*:401, July 1976.

529. Zborowski, M.: Cultural components in responses to pain. J. Soc. Issues, *8*:16, 1952.

530. Resse, E.: *The Analysis of Human Operant Behavior.* Dubuque, Iowa: William C. Brown Co., 1966.

531. Fordyce, W. E., et al.: Operant conditioning in the treatment of chronic pain. Arch. Phys. Med. Rehabil., *54*:399, Sept. 1973.

532. Basmajian, J. V., Simard, T. G.: Effects of distracting movement on the control of trained motor units. Am. J. Phys. Med., *46*:1427, Dec. 1967.

533. Green, E. E., Walters, E. D., Green, A. M., et al.: Feedback technique for deep relaxation. Psychophysiology, *6*:371, Nov. 1969.

534. Budzynski, T. H., Stoyva, J. M.: An instrument for producing deep muscle relaxation by means of analog information feedback. J. Appl. Behav. Anal., *2*:231, 1969.

535. Jacobs, A., Felton, G. S.: Visual feedback of myoelectric output to facilitate muscle relaxation in normal persons and patients with neck injuries. Arch. Phys. Med., *50*:34, Jan. 1969.

536. Fowler, R. S., Jr., Kraft, G. H.: Tension perception in patients having pain associated with chronic muscle tension. Arch. Phys. Med., *55*:28, Jan. 1974.

537. Emery, H., Schaller, J. G., Fowler, R. S., Jr.: Biofeedback in the management of primary and secondary Raynaud's. American Rheumatism Association, 40th Annual Meeting, Chicago, June, 1976. P. 77.

538. Dimond, E. G.: Acupuncture anesthesia. Western medicine and Chinese traditional medicine. JAMA, *218*:1558, 1971.

539. Bonica, J. J.: Acupuncture anesthesia in the People's Republic of China. Implications for American medicine. JAMA, *229*:1317, Sep. 1974.

540. Man, S. C., Baragar, F. D.: Preliminary clinical study of acupuncture in rheumatoid arthritis. J. Rheumatol., *1*:126, Mar. 1974.

541. Matsumoto, T., Levy, B., Ambruso, V.: Clinical evaluation of acupuncture. Am. Surg., *40*:400, July 1974.

542. Lee, P. K., et al.: Treatment of chronic pain with acupuncture. JAMA, *232*:1133, 1975.

543. Gaw, A. C., Chang, L. W., Shaw, L. C.: Efficacy of acupuncture on osteoarthritic pain. A controlled, double-blind study. N. Engl. J. Med., *293*:375, Aug. 1975.

544. Moore, M. E., Berk, S. N.: Acupuncture for chronic shoulder pain. An experimental study with attention to the role of placebo and hypnotic susceptibility. Ann. Intern. Med., *84*:381, Apr. 1976.

545. Yue, S. J., et al.: Controlled study of acupuncture for the treatment of chronic pain. Abstract presented at American Congress of Physical Medicine and Rehabilitation, Nov. 1976. P. 56.

546. Stillwell, G. K.: "Chapter 3. Clinical Electric Stimulation," *in* S. Licht, ed., *Therapeutic Electricity and Ultraviolet Radiation.* New Haven: E. Licht, 1959. Pp. 104, 133–139.

547. Millard, J. B.: The use of electrical stimulation in the rehabilitation of knee injuries. Proc. Internat. Cong. Phys. Med., London, 1952.

548. Munsat, T. L., McNeal, D., Walters, R.: Effects of nerve stimulation on human muscle. Arch. Neurol., *33*:608, Sep. 1976.

549. Fisher, S., Cleveland, S. E.: *Body Image and Personality.* Princeton, N. J.: Van Nostrand, 1958.

550. Williams, R., Krasnoff, A. G.: Bony image and physiological pattern in patients with peptic ulcer disease and rheumatoid arthritis groups. Psychosom. Med., *26*:701, 1964.

551. Rothermich, N. O., Philips, V. K.: Rheumatoid arthritis in criminal and mentally ill populations. Arthritis Rheum., *6*:639, Oct. 1963.

552. Johnson, A., Shapiro, L. B., Alexander, F.: Preliminary report on a psychosomatic study of rheumatoid arthritis. Psychosom. Med., *9*:295, Sep.–Oct. 1947.

553. Ludwig, A. O.: Psychogenic factors in rheumatoid arthritis. Bull. Rheum. Dis., *2*:15, Apr. 1952.

554. Bourestom, N. C., Howard, M. T.: Personality characteristics of three disability groups. Arch. Phys. Med. Rehabil., *46*:626, Sep. 1965.

555. Nalven, F. B., O'Brien, J. F.: On the use of the MMPI with rheumatoid arthritic patients. J. Clin. Psychol., *24*:70, Jan. 1968.

556. Solomon, G. F., Moos, R. H.: Psychologic aspects of response to treatment in rheumatoid arthritis. G.P., *32*:113, Dec. 1965.

557. Cleveland, S. E., Fisher, S.: Behavior and unconscious fantasies of patients with rheumatoid arthritis. Psychosom. Med., *16*:327, July–Aug. 1954.

558. King, S. H.: Psychosocial factors associated with rheumatoid arthritis; an evaluation of the literature. J. Chronic Dis., *2*:287, Sep. 1955.

559. Maudsley, H.: "Chapter 25. Psychophysiological autonomic and visceral disorders," *in* L. C. Kolb, ed., *Modern Clinical Psychiatry.* 8th Ed. Philadelphia: W. B. Saunders Co., 1973.

560. Engel, G. L.: "Psychogenic" pain and the pain-prone patient. Am. J. Med., June 1959. P. 899.

561. Kasl, S. V., Cobb, S.: Effects of parental status incongruence and discrepancy on physical and mental health of adult offspring. J. Personality and Social Psychol. Monograph, 7:1, 1967.

562. Wolff, B. B.: Current psychosocial concepts in rheumatoid arthritis. Bull. Rheum. Dis., *22*:656, Series 1971–72.

563. Alexander, F.: *Psychosomatic Medicine: Its Principles and Applications.* New York: W. W. Norton, 1950.

564. King, S. H., Cobb, S.: Psychosocial factors in the epidemiology of rheumatoid arthritis. J. Chronic Dis., 7:466, June 1958.

565. Freedman, A. M., Kaplan, H. I., Sadock, B. J.: *Comprehensive Textbook of Psychiatry, Vol. 2.* 2nd Ed. Baltimore: Williams & Wilkins, 1975. P. 9.

566. Geist, H.: *The Psychological Aspects of Rheumatoid Arthritis.* Springfield, Ill.: Charles C Thomas, 1966. Pp. 11, 29.

567. Vignos, P. J., Jr.: "Psycho-social problems in management of chronic arthritis," *in* G. E. Ehrlich, ed., *Total Management of the Arthritic Patient.* Philadelphia: J. B. Lippincott Co., 1973.

568. Rosillo, R. H., Fogel, M. L.: Pain, affects and progress in physical rehabilitation. J. Psychosom. Res., *17*:21, Jan. 1973.

569. Sternbach, R. A., Timmermans, G.: Personality changes associated with reduction of pain. Pain, *1*:177, 1975.

570. Wright, V., Owen, S.: The effect of rheumatoid arthritis on the social situation of housewives. Rheum. Rehabil., *15*:156, 1976.

571. Meyerowitz, S., Jacob, R. F., Hess, D. W.: Monozygotic twins discordant for rheumatoid arthritis: a genetic, clinical and psychological study of 8 sets. Arthritis Rheum., *11*:1, Feb. 1968.

572. Moldofsky, H., Rothman, A.: Personality, disease parameters, and medication in rheumatoid arthritis. Arthritis Rheum., *13*:338, May–Jun. 1970.

573. Fessel, W. J.: *Rheumatology for Clinicians.* New York: Stratton Intercontinental Medical Book Corp., 1975. P. 38.

574. Williams, R. C.: "Chapter 16. Psychiatric and Psychosocial Aspects of Rheumatoid Arthritis," *in Rheumatoid Arthritis as a Systemic Disease.* Philadelphia: W. B. Saunders Co., 1974. P. 218.

575. Freedman, A. M., Kaplan, H. I., Sadock, B. J.: *Comprehensive Textbook of Psychiatry, Vol. 2.* 2nd Ed. Baltimore: Williams & Wilkins, 1975. Pp. 1694–1704.

576. Baker, M.: Psychopathology in systemic lupus erythematosus. I. Psychiatric Observations. Semin. Arthritis Rheum., *3*:95, 1973.

577. Moos, R. H., Solomon, G. F.: Minnesota multiphasic personality inventory response patterns in patients with rheumatoid arthritis. J. Psychosom. Res., *8*:17, July 1964.

578. Cobb, S., et al.: The intrafamilial transmission of rheumatoid arthritis: an unusual study. J. Chronic Dis., *22*:193, Sep. 1969.

579. Crown, S., Crown, J. M., Fleming, A.: Aspects of the psychology of rheumatoid disease. Rheum. Rehabil., *13*:167, Nov. 1974.

580. Moos, R. H., Solomon, G. F.: Psychologic comparisons between women with rheumatoid arthritis and their non-arthritic sisters. I. Personality test and interview rating data. Psychosom. Med., *27*:135, Mar.–Apr. 1965.

581. Kutner, B.: "The Social Psychology of Disability," *in* W. S. Neff, ed., *Rehabilitation Psychology.* Washington, D.C.: American Psychiatric Association, Inc., 1971. P. 143.

582. Meyerowitz, S.: "Chapter 7. The Continuing Investigation of Psychosocial Variables in Rheumatoid Arthritis," *in* A. G. S. Hill, ed., *Modern Trends in Rheumatology —* 2. Butterworth, London, 1971.

583. Lipowski, Z. J.: Psychosocial aspects of disease. Ann. Intern. Med., *71*:1197, Dec. 1969.

584. Carnevali, D., Brueckner, S.: Immobilization — reassessment of a concept. Amer. J. Nurs., *70*:1502, July 1970.

585. Courtney, J., Davis, J. M., Solomon, P.: Sensory deprivation: the role of movement. Percept. Mot. Skills, *13*:191, 1961.

586. Zuckerman, M., Persky, H., Link, K. E., et al.: Responses to confinement: an investigation of sensory deprivation, social isolation, restriction of movement and set factors. Percept. Motor Skills, *27*:319, Aug. 1968.

587. Fabrega, H., Jr., Van Egeren, L.: A behavioral framework for the study of human disease. Ann. Internal Med., *84*:200, 1976.

588. Parsons, T., Fox, R.: Illness, therapy and the modern urban American family. J. Soc. Issues, *8*:31, 1952.

589. Mechanic, D.: The concept of illness behavior. J. Chron. Dis., *15*:189, Feb. 1952.

590. Miller, R. H., Keith, R. A.: Behavioral mapping in a rehabilitation hospital. Rehab. Psych., *20*:148, 1973.

591. Wiltse, L. L., Rocchio, P. D.: Predicting success of low back surgery by the use of preoperative psychological tests. Presented at Annual Meeting of American Orthopedic Association, Hot Springs, Virginia, June 1973.

592. Walters, J. A.: Psychogenic regional pain alias hysterical pain. Presidential address to the 11th Annual Meeting of the Canadian Neurological Society, London, July 1959.

593. Beals, R. K., Hickman, N. W.: Industrial injuries of the back and extremities.

Comprehensive evaluation — An aid in prognosis and management. A study of one hundred and eighty patients. J. Bone Joint Surg., *54A*:1593, Dec. 1972.

594. Szasz, T. R.: "The Psychology of Persistent Pain. A Portrait of L'Homme-Douloureaux," *in* A. J. Soulairac, et al., eds., *International Symposium on Pain.* New York: Academic Press, 1968. Pp. 93–113.

595. Sternbach, R. A.: *Pain; a Psychophysiological Analysis.* New York: Academic Press, 1968.

596. Clawson, D. D., Bonica, J. J., Fordyce, W. E.: "Management of chronic orthopaedic pain problems," *in* American Academy of Orthopaedic Surgeons Instructional Course Lectures, *21*:8, 1972.

597. Fordyce, W. E.: Operant conditioning as a treatment method in management of selected chronic pain problems. Northwest Med., *69*:580, Aug. 1970.

598. Grabias, S.: Topographical pain representations in the evaluation of low back pain. Resident paper presented at Rancho Los Amigos Hospital, Downey, Calif. March 29, 1974.

599. Walters, A.: "Chapter 34. The Psychogenic Regional Pain Syndrome and Its Diagnosis," *in* Knighton & Burke, eds., *Pain.* Little, Brown and Co., Inc., 1965.

600. Holmes, T. H., Rahe, R. H.: The social readjustment rating scale. J. Psychosom. Res., *11*:213, Aug. 1967.

601. Holmes, T., Masuda, M.: Psychosomatic syndrome. *Psychology Today,* April 1972.

602. Wolkind, S. N., Forrest, A. J.: Low back pain: a psychiatric investigation. Postgrad. Med. J., *48*:76, Feb. 1972.

603. Gilchrist, I. C.: Psychiatric and social factors related to low-back pain in general practice. Rheum. Rehabil., *15*:101, May 1976.

604. Maruta, T., Swanson, D. W., Swenson, W. M.: Low back pain patients in a psychiatric population. Mayo Clin. Proc., *51*:57, Jan. 1976.

605. Fordyce, W. E.: "Behavioral methods in rehabilitation," *in* W. Neff, ed., *Rehabilitation Psychology.* Washington, D.C.: American Psychological Association, 1971. Pp. 74–108.

606. Currey, H. L. F.: Osteoarthritis of the hip joint and sexual activity. Ann. Rheum. Dis., *29*:488, 1970.

607. Ehrlich, G. E.: "Chapter 9. Sexual problems of the arthritic patient," *in* G. E. Ehrlich, ed., *Total Management of the Arthritic Patient.* Philadelphia: J. B. Lippincott Co., 1973. P. 193.

608. Golden, J. S.: Sexuality and the chronically ill. The Pharos, *38*:76, 1975.

609. Carpenter, J. O.: Changing roles and disagreement in families with disabled husbands. Arch. Phys. Med. Rehabil., *55*:272, June 1974.

610. Teal, J. C., Athelstan, G. T.: Sexuality and spinal cord injury: some psychosocial considerations. Arch. Phys. Med. Rehabil., *56*:264, June 1975.

611. Griffith, E. R., Trieschmann, R. B.: Sexual functioning in women with spinal cord injury. Arch. Phys. Med. Rehabil., *56*:18, Jan. 1975.

612. Greengross, W.: *Marriage, Sex and Arthritis.* London: The Arthritis & Rheumatism Council, S. G. Beaumont, Mill Lane, Harbeldown, Canterbury, Kent.

613. Zimmerman, D.: *Sex can help arthritis.* New York: Penthouse Magazine, Nov. 1975.

614. Henkle, C.: Social group work as a treatment modality for hospitalized people with rheumatoid arthritis. Rehabil. Lit., *36*:334, Nov. 1975.

615. Mann, W., Godfrey, M. E., Dowd, E. T.: The use of group counseling procedures in the rehabilitation of spinal cord injured patients. Am. J. Occup. Therapy, *27*:73, Mar. 1973.

616. Weitz, G. W., D'Afflitti, J. G.: Rehabilitating the stroke patient through patient-family groups. Int. J. Group Psychother., *24*:323, July 1974.

617. Bouchard, V. C.: Hemiplegic exercise and discussion group. Am. J. Occup. Ther., *26*:7, 1972.

618. Sternbach, R. A.: *Pain Patients: Traits and Treatment.* New York: Academic Press, 1974. P. 105.

619. Fortin, J. N., Abse, D. W.: Group psychotherapy with peptic ulcer. Inter. J. Group Psychotherapy, *6*:383, 1956.

620. Groen, J. J., Pelser, H. E.: Experiences with and results of group psychotherapy in patients with bronchial asthma. J. Psychosom., *4*:191, 1960.

621. Rahe, R. H., O'Neil, T., Hagan, A., et al.: Brief group therapy following myocardial infarction: eighteen month follow-up of a controlled trial. Int. J. Psychiatry in Med., *6*:349, 1975.

622. Freedman, A. M., Kaplan, H. I., Sadock, B. J.: *Comprehensive Textbook of Psychiatry, Vol. 2.* 2nd Ed. Baltimore: Williams & Wilkins, 1975. P. 1858.

623. Katz, S., et al.: *Effects of continued care: Study of chronic illness in home.* Washington, D.C., U. S. Government Printing Office, Department of HEW, Publication No. (HSM) 73-3010, 1972.

624. Cauffman, J. G., Lloyd, J. S., Lyons, M. L., et al.: A study of health referral patterns. Amer. J. Public Health, *64*:331, Apr. 1974.

625. Cauffman, J.: *Inventory of Human Services (Medical and Social).* 3rd Ed. SEARCH Advisory Board of Los Angeles County, J. Cauffman, 1972.

626. Weed, L.: *Medical Records, Medical Education, and Patient Care.* Cleveland: The Press of Case Western Reserve University, 1969.

627. Swezey, R. L., Swezey, A. M.: Educational theory as a basis for patient education. J. Chronic Dis., *29*:417, July 1976.

628. Swezey, R. L.: Helping your patient live with arthritis. Med. Opinion, *9*:18, 1975.

629. Blackwell, B.: Drug therapy: Patient compliance. N. Engl. J. Med., *289*:249, Aug. 1973.

630. Ausubel, D. P.: *Educational Psychology: A Cognitive View.* New York: Holt, Rinehart and Winston, 1968.

631. Bandura, A.: *Principles of Behavior Modification.* New York: Holt, Rinehart and Winston, 1969.

632. Thorndike, E. L.: *Animal Intelligence: Experimental Studies.* Facsimile of 1911 Edition. New York: Hafner Publishing Co. 1965.

633. Skinner, B. F.: *The Behavior of Organisms.* New York: Appleton-Century-Crofts, 1938.

634. Gagné, R. M.: *The Conditions of Learning.* New York: Holt, Rinehart and Winston, 1970.

635. Hull, C. L.: *Principles of Behavior.* New York: Appleton-Century-Crofts, 1943.

636. Hebb, D. O.:*The Organization of Behavior. A Neuropsychological Theory.* New York: John Wiley, 1949.

637. Bruner, J. S.: The act of discovery. Harvard Educ. Rev., *31*:21, 1961.

638. Bloom, B. S.: *Taxonomy of Educational Objectives.* The classification of educational goals, by a committee of college and university examiners. New York: David McKay, 1956.

639. Tyler, R. W.: *Basic Principles of Curriculum and Instruction, Syllabus for Education.* Chicago: University of Chicago Press, 1950.

640. Skinner, B. F.: *The Technology of Teaching.* New York: Appleton-Century-Crofts, 1968.

641. Maslow, A. H.: *Toward a Psychology of Being.* Princeton, N. J.: Van Nostrand, 1962.

642 Davis, M. S.: Variations in patients' compliance with doctors' advice: An empirical analysis of patterns of communication. Amer. J. Public Health, *58*:274, Feb. 1968.

643. Knutson, A.: *The Individual, Society and Health Behavior.* New York: Russell Sage Foundation, 1965.

644. The Arthritis Foundation, Atlanta, Georgia.

645. Canadian Arthritis and Rheumatism Society, Toronto, Canada.

646. Klinger, J. L.: *Self-Help Manual for Arthritic Patients.* New York: Allied Health Professions Section of the Arthritis Foundation, 1974.

647. Swezey, A. M., Kaufman, A.: A model patient information library on wheels. Hospitals, 51(17):65, Sept. 1, 1977.

648. Hogsett, S. G.:*Airline Transportation for the Handicapped and Disabled.* Chicago: National Easter Seal Society, 1972.

649. Annand, D. R.: *The Wheelchair Traveler.* Milford, New Hampshire: D. R. Annand, 1974.

650. Harsanyi, S. L.: Toward equal opportunities in recreation for the disabled. Arch. Phys. Med. Rehabil., *56*:135, 1975.

651. Dunton, W. R., Jr., Licht, S.: *Occupational Therapy, Principles and Practices.* 2nd Ed. Springfield, Ill.: Charles C Thomas. 1957. P. 37.

652. Dudish, L. T.: "Starting a recreation program with limited funding in nursing homes," *in* F. M. Robinson, ed., *Therapeutic Re-Creation, Ideas and Experiences.* Springfield, Ill.: Charles C Thomas, 1974.

INDEX

Page numbers in *italics* indicate illustrations; (t) indicates table.